KU-535-660

Management of Crohn's Disease

Disease

Emma R Greig

and

David S Rampton

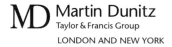
Martin Dunitz
Taylor & Francis Group
LONDON AND NEW YORK

Coventry University

© 2003 Martin Dunitz, an imprint of the Taylor & Francis Group

First published in the United Kingdom in 2003
by Martin Dunitz, an imprint of the Taylor and Francis Group, 11 New Fetter Lane,
London EC4P 4EE

Tel.:   +44 (0) 20 7583 9855
Fax.:   +44 (0) 20 7842 2298
E-mail: info@dunitz.co.uk
Website: http://www.dunitz.co.uk

All rights reserved. No part of this publication may be reproduced, stored in a retrieval
system, or transmitted, in any form or by any means, electronic, mechanical, photo-
copying, recording, or otherwise, without the prior permission of the publisher or in
accordance with the provisions of the Copyright, Designs and Patents Act 1988 or
under the terms of any licence permitting limited copying issued by the Copyright
Licensing Agency, 90 Tottenham Court Road, London W1P 0LP.

Although every effort has been made to ensure that all owners of copyright material
have been acknowledged in this publication, we would be glad to acknowledge in subsequent reprints or editions any omissions brought to our attention.

Although every effort has been made to ensure that drug doses and other information
are presented accurately in this publication, the ultimate responsibility rests with the
prescribing physician. Neither the publishers nor the authors can be held responsible
for errors or for any consequences arising from the use of information contained
herein. For detailed prescribing information or instructions on the use of any product
or procedure discussed herein, please consult the prescribing information or instruc-
tional material issued by the manufacturer.

A CIP record for this book is available from the British Library.

ISBN 1 84184 086 6

Distributed in the USA by
Fulfilment Center
Taylor & Francis
10650 Tobben Drive
Independence, KY 41051, USA
Toll Free Tel.:   +1 800 634 7064
E-mail: taylorandfrancis@thomsonlearning.com

Distributed in Canada by
Taylor & Francis
74 Rolark Drive
Scarborough, Ontario M1R 4G2, Canada
Toll Free Tel.:   +1 877 226 2237
E-mail: tal_fran@istar.ca

Distributed in the rest of the world by
Thomson Publishing Services
Cheriton House
North Way   -
Andover, Hampshire SP10 5BE, UK
Tel.:   +44 (0)1264 332424
E-mail: salesorder.tandf@thomsonpublishingservices.co.uk

Composition by Wearset Ltd, Boldon, Tyne and Wear
Printed and bound in Great Britain by The Cromwell Press Ltd

Contents

Preface

Over recent decades, the incidence of Crohn's disease in the Western world has steadily increased and it now represents a substantial burden of sickness not only in hospital clinics and wards, but also in the community. This fact, together with the major advances in treatment which have been introduced in recent years, has prompted us to attempt a practical and up-to-date text on the management of Crohn's.

In this book, a brief outline of its aetiopathogenesis, natural history, presentation and investigations will be followed by a detailed account of the medical, surgical and nutritional treatments of Crohn's disease and its physical and psychosocial complications. Separate chapters are included about the management of Crohn's disease in pregnancy and childhood. The final chapter covers the organization of care of patients with Crohn's disease in the community.

Where necessary, reference will be made to ulcerative colitis and other inflammatory disorders of the bowel, but our primary aim is to distil the rapidly burgeoning literature about Crohn's disease itself into a succinct and evidence-based guide to its management.

The book is intended principally for hospital doctors. Generalists who see patients with Crohn's disease and medical and surgical gastroenterologists in training will probably find it more useful than experienced specialists with a particular interest in inflammatory bowel disease (IBD). We hope that other professionals, such as general practitioners, specialist nurses, stoma therapists and dieticians, as well as medical students, may also find it helpful.

We would like to thank Nick Croft and Gunju Ogunbiyi for their chapters on paediatric Crohn's disease and surgical management. Furthermore, we are grateful for the assistance and patience of Alan Burgess, Robert Peden and

Abigail Griffin at Martin Dunitz and to Trudie Beason for typing some of the manuscript. We acknowledge Health Press Ltd, Oxford, for permission to reproduce Figures 2.1, 2.4, 2.6, 3.3 and 2.5 (which was provided by Dr RM Feakins, Barts and the London NHS Trust). Finally, we thank radiologists from Guy's and St Thomas' Hospital NHS Trust for the following figures: Dr AJ Saunders (Figures 2.7 and 2.9); Dr S Rankin (Figure 2.8); Dr S Vijaynathan (Figure 2.10); Dr JL Hughes (Figure 2.11) and Dr G Rottenberg (Figure 2.12).

ERG and DSR

March 2003

Contributors

Emma R Greig PhD MRCP
Specialist Registrar in Gastroenterology
Barts and The London NHS Trust
London, UK

David S Rampton DPhil FRCP
Professor of Clinical Gastroenterology
Barts and The London, Queen Mary School of Dentistry
London, UK

Nicholas M Croft PhD FRCPCH
Senior Lecturer in Paediatric Gastroenterology
Barts and The London, Queen Mary School of Medicine and Dentistry
London, UK

Olagunju A Ogunbiyi MD FRCS
Senior Lecturer/Consultant Colorectal Surgeon
Royal Free and University College Medical School
Royal Free Hospital
London, UK

chapter 1

Aetiopathogenesis of Crohn's disease

Introduction

Although the cause of Crohn's disease remains unknown, increasing evidence suggests that it results from a genetically determined inappropriately severe and/or prolonged mucosal inflammatory response to as yet unidentified enteric microbial and/or dietary factor(s) (Figure 1.1). In this chapter, the epidemiology, possible causes, pathogenesis and pathology of Crohn's disease will be outlined briefly. We shall concentrate on those aspects of

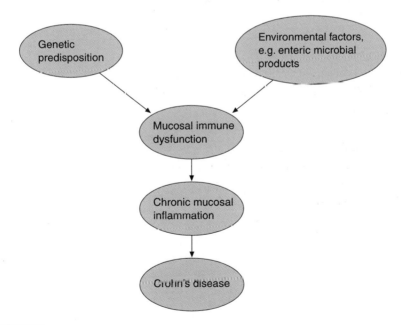

Figure 1.1 *Overview of aetiopathogenesis of Crohn's disease.*

aetiopathogenesis which have therapeutic implications, and minimize reference to animal studies.

Epidemiology

Both Crohn's disease and ulcerative colitis (UC) are more common in the Western world than in Africa, Asia or South America, and in the north of Europe than in the south.[1] In the West, the incidence of Crohn's disease has risen over the past 40 years, although it may now have levelled off (Table 1.1):[2] this increase in incidence must be explained by environmental rather than genetic factors. Inflammatory bowel disease (IBD) seems to become more common in the Third World as countries become more westernized, possibly as a result of enhanced sanitation, vaccination and increased age at exposure to enteric infections.[3,4]

Both Crohn's and UC are slightly more common in women than men and show a bimodal age distribution with a major peak at 20–30 years of age and a lesser one at 60–80. Jewish, Chinese and Asian people resident in the USA, Canada and UK are more often affected by IBD than those living in Israel, Hong Kong and Asia, respectively, indicating again the importance of environmental factors in its causation.[5,6]

Causes

Genetic and other predisposing environmental factors may differ in Crohn's disease and UC (Tables 1.2 and 1.3).

Genetic factors (Table 1.2)

Crohn's and UC are likely to be related, heterogeneous, polygenic disorders and there is no single Mendelian pattern of inheritance. The genetics of IBD are currently under intense investigation: its clarification will have major implications for our understanding of the aetiopathogenesis and for improving the treatment of IBD.[693] Genetic factors appear to be more important in Crohn's disease than in UC.

Ethnic and familial factors

IBD is more common in Ashkenazi than Sephardic Jews and in North American whites than blacks. While there is a 10-fold increased risk of IBD in the

Table 1.1 Incidence and prevalence of IBD in the Western world.[1,2]

	Crohn's disease	Ulcerative colitis
Incidence (new cases/100 000 population/year)	3–15	10
Prevalence (cases/100 000 population)	26–200	150

Table 1.2 Genetic factors in the aetiology of IBD.

Factor	Crohn's disease	Ulcerative colitis
Epidemiology		
Prevalence in first-degree relatives	10%	5%
Concordance in monozygotic twins	40%	10%
Ethnic differences in prevalence	Yes	Yes
Disease associations (e.g. ankylosing spondylitis, Turner's syndrome)	Yes	Yes
Genetic abnormalities		
HLA-DR2	—	Increased (Japanese)
Susceptibility loci		
Chromosome 16q12 (*IBD1*, *NOD2*, *CARD15*)	Yes	—
Chromosome 5q31 (*IBD5*)	Yes	—
Chromosome 14q11 (*IBD4*)	Yes	—
Chromosome 6p13 (*IBD3*)	Yes	—
Chromosome 3p21	Yes	—
Chromosome 2	—	Yes
Chromosome 12q (*IBD2*)	—	Yes
Chromosomes 1, 3, 4, 7	Yes	Yes
Gene products and markers		
Increased gut permeability	Yes	Yes
Defective colonic mucus	—	Yes
Abnormal immune regulation	Yes	Yes
pANCA	—	Yes
ASCA	Yes	—

pANCA, perinuclear antineutrophil cytoplasmic antibody.
ASCA, antisaccharomyces cerevisiae antibody.

Table 1.3 Possible environmental disease-modifying factors in Crohn's disease.

Smoking
Diet*
Microbiological factors
  Enteric flora
  *Mycobacterium paratuberculosis**
  Measles*
  MMR*
Drugs
  NSAIDs
  Antibiotics
  Oral contraceptive pill
Stress*

---

* Evidence contentious.
MMR, measles–mumps–rubella vaccination.
NSAID, non-steroidal anti-inflammatory drug.

first-degree relatives of patients with UC, the risk is even higher (15–40-fold) for relatives of patients with Crohn's.[7] There is a high rate of concordance for IBD in monozygotic twins, again particularly in Crohn's (40%) as opposed to UC (<10%).[8]

Genetic studies

The results of genetic studies have varied according to the population under investigation. However, in several populations, susceptibility loci have been reported for Crohn's disease at the pericentromeric region of chromosome 16 (*IBD1*)[9] and on chromosomes 3, 5 (*IBD5*), 6 (*IBD3*), 12 (*IBD2*) and 14 (*IBD4*) (Table 1.2).[10,11]

IBD1, NOD2 (*CARD 15*) gene

Two single nucleotide polymorphisms and one frame-shift mutation of the *NOD2* (recently renamed caspase-activating recruitment domain, *CARD 15*) gene at the *IBD1* locus on chromosome 16 have recently been reported to be associated with Crohn's disease.[9,12] The risk of Crohn's was increased over 40-fold for individuals homozygous for all three polymorphisms.[9]

Conversely, about 40% of European patients with familial Crohn's disease carry one of the three *NOD2* mutations.[9] Early reports indicate that *NOD2* mutations predispose particularly to fibrostenosing ileal and right-sided colonic Crohn's disease.[13,14]

One of the polymorphisms identified may confer susceptibility to Crohn's disease by altering recognition by monocytes of microbial pathogens and/or by increasing activation of the pro-inflammatory nuclear transcription factor, NFkβ (see below).[9] In contrast, another polymorphism appears to inhibit activation of NFkβ by bacterial lipopolysaccharide (LPS),[12] leading to an abnormal adaptive response to enteric bacteria. Other potential pathogenic effects of the mutations include alterations in apoptosis and reduced production of anti-inflammatory cytokines.[10,15]

Other gene products and genetic markers

How the other chromosomal susceptibility loci so far identified might influence the pathogenesis and/or phenotype of IBD is not yet known. However, definition of the genetic abnormalities underlying Crohn's disease is likely in due course to increase diagnostic accuracy and efficiency, clarify and enable prediction of disease phenotype, facilitate family counselling and make possible forecasting of therapeutic response in individual patients (see Chapters 3 and 6).

pANCA and ASCA

The presence of perinuclear antineutrophil cytoplasmic antibodies (pANCA) in the serum of 50–80% of patients with UC, as against only about 10% of those with Crohn's, is likely to be determined genetically.[16,17] The same may apply to the converse finding of antibodies to *Saccharomyces cerevisiae* (ASCA) in about 60% of patients with Crohn's disease, as opposed to only 5% of those with UC.[18] In Crohn's, the presence of high titres of ASCA appears to be associated with early age of onset, and both fibrostenosing and internally penetrating rather than other types of disease behaviour.[19]

Environmental factors

Since the concordance rate for Crohn's disease in monozygotic twins is only 40% (Table 1.2), the environment must play a major role in its pathogenesis. Epidemiological and other evidence has identified a number of potentially important environmental factors (Table 1.3).

Smoking

It is an unexplained but intriguing observation that only about 10% of patients with UC smoke, compared with 30% of the normal population and 40% of those with Crohn's disease.[20] Indeed, in siblings who have a similar genetic predisposition to IBD, those who smoke tend to develop Crohn's disease, while non-smokers get ulcerative colitis.[21] Smoking in Crohn's increases the risks of relapse, of the need for immunosuppressive therapy and of surgery, especially in women.[22,23] Furthermore, patients who stop smoking do better than those who continue.[24]

Nicotine and other constituents of tobacco smoke have a variety of effects on the inflammatory response,[20] but it is not known why these are harmful in patients with Crohn's but beneficial in those with UC.

Diet

Patients with active Crohn's improve on replacement of ordinary food by a liquid formula diet,[25,26] and have been reported thereafter to deteriorate on the introduction of specific foods (Chapters 5 and 6).[27] Proposed dietary triggers include particles such as titanium oxide and aluminosilicates, fluoride and cornflakes, but none has yet been substantiated.[28,29] Although no individual foods universally detrimental to patients with Crohn's have been identified, it is conceivable that some foods may prove pathogenic, through direct adverse effects on mucosal immunity or by modifying luminal gut flora (see below).

Specific infection

Epidemiological, molecular biological and/or pharmacological studies have suggested initiating roles for *Mycobacterium paratuberculosis*[30] and measles virus and vaccination[31,32] in the pathogenesis of Crohn's disease, but available data are controversial. In neither instance have Koch's postulates been fulfilled and more work is needed to elucidate the possible roles of each of these organisms in Crohn's disease.

Enteric microflora

The resident gut microflora are complex and dynamic, and likely to be a major environmental factor in the pathogenesis of both Crohn's disease and UC.[6,15] The normal flora influence the function of the mucosal immune system and also have effects on epithelial turnover, mucus secretion, mucosal blood flow and peristalsis.[33] Human clinical and experimental evidence showing the importance of the faecal stream in driving mucosal inflammation in Crohn's disease is summarized in Table 1.4.

Drugs

Relapse of IBD may be precipitated by non-steroidal anti-inflammatory drugs (NSAIDs), perhaps as a result of inhibition of the synthesis of cytoprotective prostaglandins,[34–36] and occasionally by antibiotics, possibly secondary to adverse changes in enteric flora.[37]

The oral contraceptive pill has also been associated epidemiologically with Crohn's disease (Chapter 7), the risk being associated with duration of usage but not the oestrogen content of the preparation.[38]

Stress

For many years, IBD was thought to be a psychosomatic disorder. This theory has now been discredited,[39] because more recent studies have shown that most patients with Crohn's disease and UC are psychologically normal. One study has suggested that patients with Crohn's are more extrovert than those with UC,[40] but in general psychiatric disorders in IBD are less common than in irritable bowel syndrome.[41]

Although animal studies support the concept that stress may worsen IBD,[42] and many patients and their doctors are convinced that stress can provoke relapse, the literature to date does not confirm this.[43,44] Furthermore, there are no trials to show that treatment or removal of stress is therapeutically helpful (Chapter 9).

Psychological stress is common in patients with Crohn's, as a result of the unpleasantness, chronicity and intractability of their illness. It is possible, moreover, that in some patients, as in animal models, stress itself triggers relapse by activation of lymphocytes by enteric nerve endings (Figure 1.2).[6]

Table 1.4 Evidence that gut bacterial flora drive mucosal inflammation in Crohn's disease.

Patients with Crohn's disease show:
- Inflammatory lesions where flora are most abundant
- Loss of immunological tolerance to gut flora
- Mucosal antibodies to gut flora
- Abnormalities of faecal and mucosa-associated flora
- Response to diversion of the faecal stream
- Response to antibiotics and possibly probiotics

Pathogenesis

Although its precise initiating factors are unknown, Crohn's disease is characterized by a loss of mucosal immune tolerance so that instead of down-regulating the inflammatory response to luminal antigens, antigen-presenting cells such as dendritic cells and macrophages secrete a profile of cytokines which lead to a prolonged and excessive mucosal inflammatory response; this, in turn, is amplified and perpetuated by recruitment of leuko-cytes from the gut vasculature.[6,45] In Crohn's disease, a Th1-induced cell-mediated response predominates, while in UC a non-Th1 cytokine response

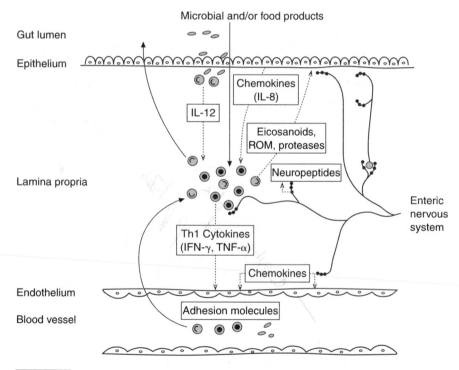

Figure 1.2 *Schematic representation of cross-section of intestinal mucosa showing proposed steps in the pathogenesis of Crohn's disease. Although the initiating factor(s) are uncertain, they are likely to include a breakdown in tolerance to enteric flora, leading to activation of T-cells and macrophages with production of a range of pro-inflammatory cytokines. Cytokine-driven recruitment and activation of further inflammatory cells leads to tissue damage by metalloproteases and other reactive substances, augmentation of the inflammatory response and disruption of the epithelial barrier, itself causing further ingress of enteric flora and their products. (Reproduced from Shanahan. Lancet 2002;* **359***: 62–9[6] with permission from Elsevier) IL, interleukin; ROM, reactive oxygen metabolities; IFN-γ, interferon-γ; TNF-α, tumour necrosis factor α.*

generates a largely humoral immune profile (Table 1.5).[46] Up-regulation of the expression of nuclear transcription factors such as NFκβ[47,48] is likely to underlie the subsequent release locally of further cytokines, growth factors, reactive oxygen metabolites, nitric oxide, eicosanoids, proteases, neuropeptides and other mediators (Table 1.6) (Figure 1.2).[49–51] In both forms of IBD,

Table 1.5 Immune and inflammatory response in IBD.

	Crohn's disease	*Ulcerative colitis*
Humoral immunity		
Association with auto-immune disease (Hashimoto's thyroiditis, SLE, etc.)	Weak	Strong
Autoantibody production (anticolon antibody, pANCA etc.)	Rare	Common
Cell-mediated immunity		
Mucosal infiltrate	Granulomatous; T-lymphocytes prominent	Non-granulomatous; neutrophils prominent
T-cell reactivity	Increased	Normal/decreased
Cytokine profile		
Th response	Th1 (IL-2, IFN-γ, IL-12, IL-18, TNF-β)	NonTh1 (IL-10, IL-1, IL-6, IL-8, TNF-α IL-4, IL-5, IL-13)
Other cytokines	IL-1, IL-6, TNF-α	

Th, T-helper lymphocyte; IL, interleukin; IFN, interferon; TNF, tumour necrosis factor.

Table 1.6 Principal soluble mediators involved in the pathogenesis of Crohn's disease.[49,51]

Eicosanoids	*Reactive metabolites*	*Matrix metalloproteases*
Prostaglandins	Superoxide	Stromolysin-1
Thromboxanes	Hypochlorite	
Leukotrienes	Hydroxyl ion	
	Nitric oxide	
	Peroxynitrite	

abnormal intestinal epithelial permeability may increase access of luminal dietary and bacterial products to the mucosa.[52] In Crohn's disease, a procoagulant diathesis[53] and multifocal granulomatous intestinal microinfarction may occur early in the disease process.[54]

Conclusions

Although the aetiology of Crohn's disease remains unclear, the gradual elucidation of its pathogenesis has improved our understanding of the clinical and pathological features of the disease. It has also clarified the possible modes of action of conventional treatment and has led to the development of entirely new therapeutic approaches aimed at specific pathophysiological targets (see Figure 3.5).

chapter 2

Clinical features, prognosis and diagnosis of Crohn's disease

Introduction

Crohn's disease can affect any part of the gastrointestinal tract from mouth to anus. Adults with Crohn's disease tend to present with either ileocaecal or colonic disease, with isolated small bowel disease and other presentations being less common.[55]

The frequencies of disease site for adults with Crohn's disease are shown in Table 2.1. Diffuse jejunoileal disease is disproportionately common in children and adolescents; in contrast, the incidence of colonic disease in adults increases with age.[56] These phenotypic differences are likely to be genetically determined.

The natural history of Crohn's disease is characterized by relapses occurring between spontaneous or treatment-induced remissions;[57] however, about 15% of patients have non-remitting disease and 10% prolonged remission.[2] The symptoms and signs of Crohn's depend on both its site and the predominant pathological process occurring in each patient. Symptoms may

Table 2.1 Sites of Crohn's disease in adults.[55,58]

Site	Patients (%)
Ileocolonic	45
Colitis only	25
Terminal ileum only	20
Extensive small bowel	5
Anorectal only	3
Other (gastroduodenal, oral only)	2

be of insidious onset and initially non-specific so that diagnosis may be delayed for months or years.[55,58]

In this chapter, brief descriptions of the clinical features of each of the major intestinal presentations of Crohn's disease and of its prognosis are followed by an overview of the investigations used in its management. How disease activity is assessed using clinical and laboratory measures is then outlined. The chapter concludes with an outline of the differential diagnosis of Crohn's disease, together with algorithms showing relevant diagnostic pathways.

Clinical features

Active ileocaecal Crohn's disease

This usually presents with pain and/or a tender mass in the right iliac fossa. Diarrhoea is commonly associated; its mechanisms include mucosal inflammation, bile salt malabsorption and bacterial overgrowth proximal to a stricture (Table 2.2). In patients with symptoms predominantly due to inflammation or abscess, the pain tends to be constant, often with fever. In patients with small bowel obstruction, whether due to active inflammation or to fibrosis and stricture formation, the pain is more generalized, intermittent, colicky and associated with loud borborygmi, abdominal distension, vomiting and eventually constipation. Presentation as an acute abdomen, with peritonitis due to free perforation, is rare. In patients with chronic active disease there are frequently systemic symptoms including lethargy, anorexia, weight loss, low grade fever and finger clubbing.

Table 2.2 Mechanisms of diarrhoea in Crohn's disease.[99]

Mechanism	Treatment
Inflammation	Anti-inflammatory drugs (Chapters 3 and 6)
Small bowel bacterial overgrowth	Antibiotics
Bile salt diarrhoea	Cholestyramine
Bile salt deficiency	Low-fat diet
Lactase deficiency	Avoidance of lactose
Short bowel syndrome	See Chapter 9 (short bowel syndrome)
Intestinal fistula	Surgery
Antibiotic-related	Stop antibiotics
Other disorder (irritable bowel syndrome, coeliac disease)	As appropriate

Extensive small bowel Crohn's disease

As well as the above symptoms, patients with extensive small bowel disease may have features of malabsorption, with steatorrhoea, anaemia and weight loss.

Active Crohn's colitis

Active Crohn's colitis causes diarrhoea with peri-defaecatory abdominal pain and systemic features (see above). Overt rectal bleeding is not as common as in ulcerative colitis, but occult blood loss may be sufficient to cause iron deficiency anaemia.[58] Massive rectal bleeding occurs occasionally from colonic and/or small bowel ulceration, but toxic megacolon and free perforation are rare (Chapter 4).

Fistulating Crohn's disease

Fistulae result from extension of transmural inflammation through the serosa to create a sinus tract. This may end blindly, producing an intra-abdominal or psoas abscess. Alternatively, it may penetrate into adjacent bowel loops causing an enteroenteric fistula, into the bladder (enterovesical fistula) or vagina (enterovaginal fistula). Penetration of the abdominal wall to the skin surface leads to an enterocutaneous fistula. Internal and enterocutaneous fistulae occur most commonly in patients with ileocolonic disease (approximately one-third). Enterocutaneous fistulae are clinically obvious, but direct questions about pneumaturia and faeculent vaginal discharge may be necessary to identify enterovesical and enterovaginal fistulae, respectively.

Perianal Crohn's disease

Perianal fistulae and sepsis occur in about one-third of patients with ileocolonic and one-third of those with exclusively colorectal disease.[59] They may be relatively asymptomatic or, alternatively, associated with local mucus and/or faeculent discharge, tenesmus, pruritus ani and rectal bleeding. Local pain suggests a fissure or complicating perianal abscess. Anorectal strictures are uncommon: they may be asymptomatic or associated with constipation and incontinence. Although perianal Crohn's disease is often less uncomfortable than it looks, in some patients rectal examination and sigmoidoscopy (see below) may be too painful to undertake without sedation or even anaesthesia.

Gastroduodenal Crohn's disease

Although microscopic abnormalities, in particular focal foveolar gastritis, are common in the gastric mucosa of patients with Crohn's,[694] symptomatic gastroduodenal Crohn's disease is rare.[61] It presents with upper abdominal pain or dyspepsia, often with anorexia, nausea, vomiting and weight loss.

Oesophageal Crohn's disease

Crohn's disease of the oesophagus is rare, affecting less than 1% of patients symptomatically. Presentation is with chest pain, odynophagia and dysphagia.[60]

Oral Crohn's disease

Crohn's disease may affect any part of the oral cavity. Previously rare, oral Crohn's seems to be increasing in incidence in young people. The disease causes chronic ulceration, tags, cobble-stoning and induration of the lips, oral cavity and/or tongue.[62,63] Half of patients have no other manifestations of Crohn's disease. Biopsies may show granulomas, and the condition needs to be distinguished from other granulomatous oral diseases including Melkersson–Rosenthal syndrome and sarcoidosis.[64]

Extraintestinal manifestations

These are described in Chapter 9.

Prognosis of Crohn's disease

Morbidity in patients with Crohn's disease

Most patients with Crohn's disease are able to lead a normal life, with 75% in one population-based study able to work normally.[65] However, 15–20% of patients were disabled at five years from diagnosis, compared with 4% of the general population.

Natural history

Interpretation of reports about factors influencing the natural history of Crohn's disease is compromised by the heterogeneity of the disease and by differing definitions of recurrence. Efforts to standardize disease phenotypes have recently resulted in the 'Vienna' classification system, in which three variables are treated as phenotypic endpoints: age at diagnosis, disease location and disease behaviour (non-stricturing, stricturing, non-penetrating and penetrating).[66] The largest surveys of the course of Crohn's disease (see below) were made before these criteria were published. Definitions of recurrence range from symptomatic, through endoscopic, histological or radiological recurrence, to the need for surgery and use of immunosuppressive therapy.

In relation to the effect of disease site on the natural history of Crohn's, the need for surgery and the risks of postoperative recurrence are greater in ileocolonic disease than exclusively small bowel disease.[67,68] In Farmer's study, the times to a second operation were five and nine years in patients whose initial surgical indications were perforating and non-perforating disease, respectively.[68]

Younger age at diagnosis (<20 years) is associated particularly with small bowel involvement, stricturing disease and the need for surgery. Conversely, older age at diagnosis (>40 years) is associated with colonic disease and a more benign disease course.[69]

Many of these factors are likely to be determined by the patient's genotype.[7] It already appears, for example, that *NOD2* (*CARD15*) gene mutations are linked with ileal disease, fibrostenosis and early age of onset of disease,[13,14] and the *IBD5* locus mutations with early onset.[70]

Of environmental factors, smoking is the major prognostic influence, increasing the frequency of relapse and the need for surgery and immunosuppressive therapy, particularly in women.[22–24]

Mortality in patients with Crohn's disease

Although most recent studies have shown no increase in overall mortality compared with the general population,[71–73] certain features of disease are associated with an increased risk of death from Crohn's disease. These include either young[72,73] or much older age at diagnosis, the first five years after diagnosis, small bowel disease,[71] multiple operations, smoking and female gender.[71–73] Death from Crohn's disease results from sepsis, pulmonary embolism, surgery and immunosuppressive therapy.

In addition, most studies reveal an increase in intestinal cancers.[72–74] The risk of haemolymphopoietic malignancies continues to be debated.[75]

Investigations

Introduction

The aims of investigation are to establish the diagnosis of Crohn's disease, its site and activity, and to check for complications of the disease and its treatment. The investigations which can be used are summarized in Table 2.3. The following outline of what each investigation offers will be succeeded by a section on how they are used to assess disease activity and finally in the diagnosis of patients with particular clinical presentations.

Blood tests

Haematology

In patients presenting for the first time with undiagnosed abdominal pain and/or diarrhoea, anaemia, raised platelet count and raised ESR may suggest active IBD, but are not diagnostic. Patients with extensive chronic terminal ileal Crohn's disease may have low serum B_{12}, while a low red cell folate may indicate active chronic inflammation, reduced intake or malabsorption. Iron deficiency is common, although again not diagnostic of Crohn's disease.

One of the purposes of blood tests in patients with Crohn's disease is to assess and monitor disease activity (see below). This is related directly to platelet count, ESR and C-reactive protein, and inversely to serum haemoglobin and albumin concentrations.[76] A raised neutrophil count may suggest intra-abdominal abscess, but patients already on corticosteroids for their Crohn's disease may have a leukocytosis caused by demargination of intravascular neutrophils.

Regular blood counts are used to check for bone marrow depression in patients maintained on immunosuppressive drugs such as azathioprine/6-mercaptopurine and methotrexate (Chapters 3, 6 and 10). Patients on aminosalicylates carry a very low risk of bone marrow depression but do require periodic blood counts (see Chapters 3 and 10); the rare patients now taking sulphasalazine are also at risk of haemolytic anaemia and folate deficiency.

Biochemistry

Raised C-reactive protein and low serum albumin concentrations suggest active disease in patients with established Crohn's, but are not diagnostic of IBD in those in whom the diagnosis has not yet been made. Low serum albumin, calcium, magnesium, zinc and essential fatty acid concentrations

Table 2.3 Investigations in Crohn's disease. A selective approach is advocated (see text and Figures 2.13–2.15): most patients do not require all these tests.

Blood tests	*Haematology*	Haemoglobin
		White blood cells
		Platelets
		ESR
		Ferritin
		B_{12}
		Red cell folate
	Biochemistry	C-reactive protein
		Albumin, urea and electrolytes
		Liver function tests
		Calcium, magnesium, zinc
	Serology	Anti-endomysial antibodies
		pANCA, ASCA
		Amoebiasis
		Strongyloides
		Schistosomiasis
		Human immunodeficiency virus (HIV)
Microbiological tests	*Stool*	Microscopy and culture
		Clostridium difficile toxin
	Other	Tuberculin skin testing
		Mucosal acid-fast bacilli culture
Endoscopy with biopsy		Sigmoidoscopy
		Colonoscopy
		Oesophagogastroduodenoscopy
		Enteroscopy
		Wireless capsule endoscopy
Conventional radiology		Chest and abdominal X-rays
		Barium follow-through/small bowel enema (enteroclysis)
		Fistulography
		Barium enema
Isotope scanning		^{99}Tc-HMPAO-labelled leukocyte scan
Other radiology		Ultrasound
		CT scanning
		Magnetic resonance imaging
		PET scanning

ESR, erythrocyte sedimentation rate; pANCA, anti-neutrophil cytoplasmic antibodies; ASCA, anti-saccharomyces cerevisiae antibodies; CT, computerized tomography; PET, positron emission tomography; ^{99}Tc-HMPAO, ^{99}technetium-hexamethylpropyleneamine oxine.

may be found in patients with malabsorption, while liver function tests are abnormal in patients with hepatobiliary complications of IBD (see Chapter 9) and require regular monitoring in patients on immunosuppressive therapy (see Chapters 3 and 10). Serum urea and creatinine concentrations should be checked periodically in patients taking aminosalicylates (Chapters 3 and 10).

Serology

In patients presenting for the first time with diarrhoea, coeliac disease is usually excluded by a negative test for endomysial antibodies. Circulating antibodies to *Saccharomyces cerevisiae* (ASCA) are found more frequently in Crohn's disease than in ulcerative colitis or healthy controls (see Chapter 1), but their diagnostic role has not yet been established.[77]

Microbiology

Stools

In patients with a recent onset of diarrhoea (whether a diagnosis of Crohn's disease has yet been established or not), stool samples should be sent for microscopy for ova, cysts and parasites, and for culture for bacterial pathogens including *Clostridium difficile* toxin.

Serology

Tests for *Yersinia*, amoebae, *Schistosoma* and *Strongyloides* may be useful in some patients, particularly those who have travelled abroad.

Excluding tuberculosis

Intestinal tuberculosis should be considered in patients from endemic areas, as well as in immunocompromised patients presenting with symptoms or signs suggestive of Crohn's disease. Exclusion of coexistent pulmonary tuberculosis is also essential when treatment of Crohn's disease with infliximab is being planned (see Chapters 3 and 6).

Chest X-rays and the tuberculin skin test are unfortunately abnormal in less than half of patients with intestinal tuberculosis. The mucosal appearances of Crohn's and tuberculosis on barium radiology or ileocolonoscopy (see below) are similar. Although a definitive diagnosis of tuberculosis can be made only by identification of the bacillus by microscopy or culture of involved mucosa, other features of endoscopic biopsies may be useful in distinguishing tuberculosis from Crohn's disease.[78] Polymerase chain reaction

(PCR) techniques have not yet proven sufficiently sensitive and specific for intestinal tuberculosis.[79] Abdominal CT may be helpful, however, if it shows lymphadenopathy or free peritoneal fluid, making the diagnosis more likely to be tuberculosis than Crohn's; fine needle aspiration of enlarged nodes or aspiration of ascites may confirm the diagnosis. Laparoscopy is occasionally necessary, in particular to find and biopsy peritoneal seedlings, but laparotomy with resection of diseased bowel is now rarely necessary: in indeterminate cases, a therapeutic trial with anti-tuberculous therapy for three months in the first instance is usually preferable.

Endoscopy

Ileocolonoscopy

Colonoscopy with terminal ileoscopy and biopsy is central to the diagnosis of Crohn's disease (see Chapter 6); it has largely superseded barium enema.

In early Crohn's disease, prominent lymphoid follicles (the red-ring sign) are followed by aphthoid ulceration (Figure 2.1). Later, larger pleomorphic and deep ulcers develop, separated by relatively normal-looking mucosa (Figures 2.2 and 2.3). The cobblestone appearance of the mucosa is a late sign (Figure 2.4). Fibrosis and stricturing may occur. Changes are often segmental (skip lesions).

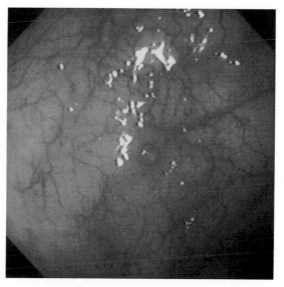

Figure 2.1 Colonoscopic view of aphthoid ulceration in sigmoid colon in early Crohn's disease. (Please see front cover for colour image.)

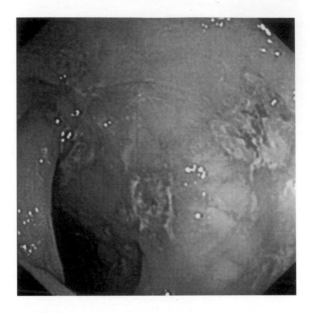

Figure 2.2 *Colonoscopic view of pleomorphic superficial ulceration in sigmoid colon in Crohn's disease. (Please see front cover for colour image.)*

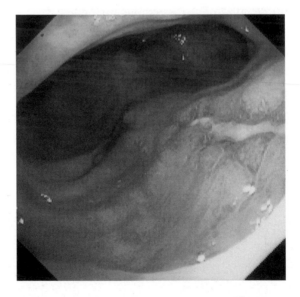

Figure 2.3 *Colonoscopic view of linear ulcer in sigmoid colon in Crohn's disease. (Please see front cover for colour image.)*

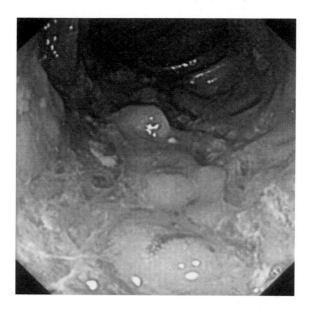

Figure 2.4 *Colonoscopic view of cobblestone mucosa with superficial ulceration in transverse colon in Crohn's disease. (Please see front cover for colour image.)*

Aphthous ulcers and rectal sparing are more common in Crohn's disease than UC but are not diagnostic.[56] Endoscopic features which may help distinguish Crohn's disease from UC are shown in Table 2.4.

In established Crohn's colitis, colonoscopy during acute relapse is not routinely necessary and may, as in UC, predispose to acute colonic dilatation and perforation. However, where there is doubt about disease activity, colonoscopy may provide crucially important information.[80]

Table 2.4 Endoscopic features helping to distinguish Crohn's disease from ulcerative colitis.

Feature	Crohn's disease	Ulcerative colitis
Rectum	Often spared	Usually involved
Inflammation	Discontinuous, asymmetric	Continuous
Ulceration	In normal mucosa	In inflamed mucosa
	Aphthoid, linear and/or serpiginous	—
Cobblestoning	Yes	—
Stricture	Sometimes	Rarely
Fistula	Occasionally	—

As in UC, colonoscopy may play a role in screening for colorectal cancer in patients with chronic Crohn's colitis (see Chapter 9).[81] Other indications include preoperative assessment of disease extent in patients with ileal disease and the early assessment of recurrence after right hemicolectomy;[82] it can also be used for balloon dilatation of terminal ileal, colorectal and anastomotic strictures (see Chapter 6, Figure 6.3).

Oesophagogastroduodenescopy (OGD) and enteroscopy

Video endoscopy of the upper GI tract is helpful diagnostically in the minority of patients with Crohn's disease affecting the oesophagus, stomach, duodenum or proximal jejunum, and for dilating strictures in these sites (see Chapter 6).

Wireless capsule endoscopy

The recent advent of wireless capsule endoscopy makes possible the non-invasive visualization of small bowel inaccessible to the conventional endoscope.[83] Use of this test for the diagnosis of Crohn's, however, may be compromised by the inability of the capsule, at present, to take biopsies (see below). Furthermore, patients with intestinal strictures are at risk of capsule-induced obstruction.

Histopathology of biopsies

Microscopic features helping to differentiate Crohn's disease from UC are shown in Table 2.5. In Crohn's disease, ileocolonoscopic biopsies

Table 2.5 Histological features of Crohn's disease and ulcerative colitis.[99]

Feature	Crohn's disease	Ulcerative colitis
Ulceration	Deep	Superficial
Goblet cell mucin depletion	Rare	Marked
Cryptitis, crypt abscesses	Focal	Prominent
Crypt distortion and loss	Patchy	Widespread
Lamina propria cell infiltrate	Discontinuous, deep; lymphocytes predominant	Diffuse, superficial; neutrophils predominant
Epithelioid granulomas	Occasional	None

characteristically show patchy transmural inflammatory cell infiltration with ulceration and microabscess formation. Non-caseating epithelioid granulomas, sometimes containing multi-nucleate giant cells, are found in biopsies of about 25% patients with Crohn's (Figure 2.5). They are not, however, diagnostic of Crohn's and may be found in several other infections (e.g. tuberculosis, schistosomiasis, yersiniosis, campylobacteriosis), in sarcoidosis, in diverticular colitis and in response to crypt rupture and foreign bodies.[84]

Imaging

Plain abdominal radiograph

Plain abdominal radiography is used to look for dilated and fluid-filled loops of bowel if intestinal obstruction is suspected (Figure 2.6). It may also hint at a mass in the right iliac fossa in patients with ileal disease. A plain film in active Crohn's colitis may show deep mucosal ulceration, thickened bowel wall and rarely colonic dilatation.[85] Sometimes, radio-opaque urinary or gall stones complicating Crohn's disease are seen.

Small bowel contrast radiology

The earliest manifestation of Crohn's disease on contrast radiology is the aphthoid ulcer. These enlarge, deepen and may form confluent serpiginous longitudinal tracks with transverse fissuring and oedematous intervening

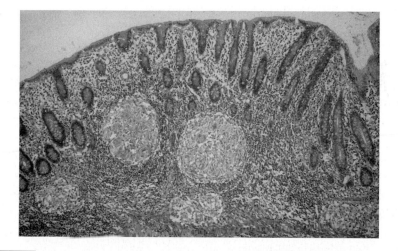

Figure 2.5 *Microscopic appearance of chronic Crohn's disease showing three large epithelioid granulomas with multi-nucleate giant cells. (Reproduced courtesy of Dr R Feakins, Barts and The London NHS Trust.) (Please see front cover for colour image.)*

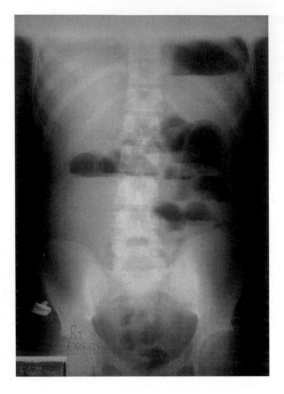

Figure 2.6 Radiological appearances on plain abdominal radiography of small intestinal obstruction.

mucosa, giving the typical cobblestone appearance (Figure 2.7). These changes tend to affect the mesenteric border of the small bowel preferentially. There is associated oedema and thickening of mucosal folds. Local inflammation may progress to stricturing (Figure 2.8), while deep ulcers may penetrate the bowel wall to cause sinuses, abscesses and fistulae into adjacent bowel, other hollow viscera or through the skin (Figure 2.9).

For imaging the small intestine, a barium follow-through is more comfortable for patients, appears less likely to miss proximal disease and is safer than a small bowel enema (enteroclysis).[86] Nevertheless, a small bowel enema may be very useful in defining strictured segments accurately in subacute small bowel obstruction, particularly if surgery is contemplated.[87]

Radiolabelled leukocyte scans
The intensity and extent of intestinal uptake one hour after injection of autologous, radiolabelled leukocytes provide information, non-invasively,

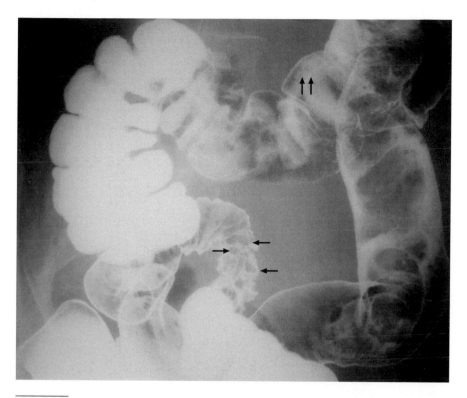

Figure 2.7 *Barium enema appearance of cobblestone mucosa and aphthous ulceration in Crohn's disease. Cobblestone mucosa seen as islands of normal mucosa (→) in the terminal ileum with intervening ulceration seen as linear tracks of barium. Aphthous ulceration is also seen in the transverse colon (↑↑). (Reproduced courtesy of Dr A Saunders, Guy's Hospital, London.)*

about disease activity and particularly extent and site, where doubt exists in patients with Crohn's disease (Figure 2.10).[88] Labelling with 99-technetium-hexamethylpropyleneamine oxine (^{99}Tc-HMPAO) is preferred to ^{111}indium because of its superior definition, lower radiation dose, shorter scanning interval and lower cost.[88] Increased isotopic activity on such scans is not specific for Crohn's disease as positive results are obtained in other inflammatory gut diseases including UC. Furthermore, both false-positive and false-negative results may occur, the latter particularly in small bowel Crohn's disease.[89]

Radiolabelled leukocyte scanning is particularly useful in symptomatic patients to discriminate active inflammatory strictures from those due to fibrosis. It can also complement ultrasound and CT where local sepsis is suspected. In patients with mucosal inflammation, delayed scans outline more

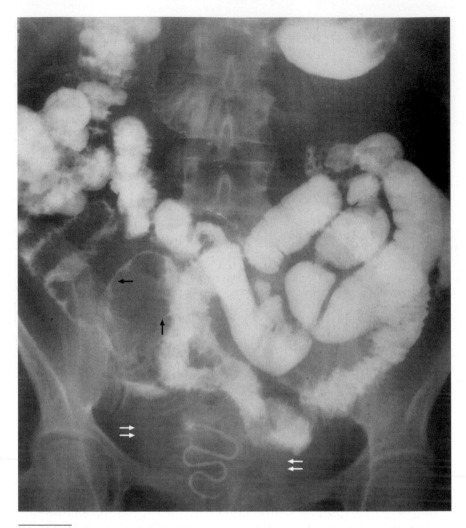

Figure 2.8 *Barium radiology appearance of stricturing disease with free perforation. Barium follow through study showing rose thorn ulcers (↑) and stricturing (←) in the terminal ileum. The head of the barium column has only reached the hepatic flexure. There is free barium in the pelvis (double white arrows outline lateral margins) due to a perforation into the peritoneal cavity. Incidentally, there is a Lippes loop intrauterine device in the pelvis. (Reproduced courtesy of Dr S Rankin, Guy's Hospital, London.)*

distal bowel as the radiolabelled leukocytes that have migrated into the lumen move distally; in patients with an abscess, the site of uptake remains constant and gradually intensifies.

Finally, the ^{75}Se-homocholic acid test (SeHCAT) isotope scan is useful for confirming bile acid malabsorption in patients with watery diarrhoea.[90]

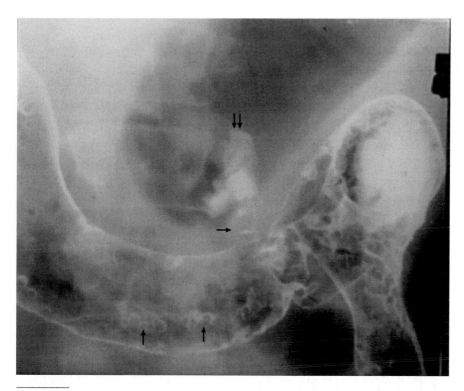

Figure 2.9 *Barium radiology appearance of gastro-colic fistula and inflammatory polyps. Double contrast barium enema showing inflammatory pseudopolyps (↑) in the transverse colon. Barium is seen in a fistulous track (→) between the superior border of the transverse colon and the stomach (seen as a gas shadow). The barium disperses in the stomach lumen (↓↓). (Reproduced courtesy of Dr A Saunders, Guy's Hospital, London.)*

Ultrasound

Transabdominal ultrasound for the assessment of bowel wall abnormalities, abscess and fistula is becoming more widespread.[86,91] Changes in mucosal and superior mesenteric arterial blood flow indicating active Crohn's disease are detectable by colour Doppler ultrasound, whereas endoanal and trans-vaginal ultrasound can help to evaluate perianal disease.[92] Although its non-invasive nature and lack of radiation exposure make ultrasound an appealing investigative technique, results are highly dependent on operator skill and equipment quality.

Abdominal CT scanning

Abdominal computed tomography (CT) now has a major role in the diagnosis of abscess, fistula and perianal and parastomal complications of Crohn's

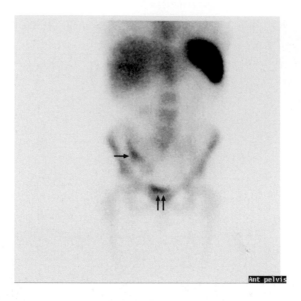

Figure 2.10 *^{99}Tc-HMPAO radiolabelled leukocyte scan showing active ileocaecal inflammation (→). ^{99}Tc-HMPAO labelled leukocyte image obtained 4 hours after injection of radio-pharmaceutical. Normal uptake is seen in the spleen and liver. In contra-distinction to ^{111}Indium scanning, excretion in the gallbladder and urinary bladder (↑↑) is normal in ^{99m}Tc HMPAO leukocyte imaging.*

disease[86] (Figure 2.11). Like ultrasound, CT also makes possible the percutaneous drainage of localized collections.

MRI scanning

The contribution of magnetic resonance imaging (MRI) to the diagnosis and management of Crohn's disease is evolving, but this technique is already invaluable for the delineation of pelvic and perianal disease (Figure 2.12).[92] Furthermore, it has recently been suggested that MRI might be superior to CT in the detection of mural abnormalities in Crohn's disease,[93] and if mural enhancement with gadolinium is sought, provides a guide to disease activity.[94]

PET scanning

Functional positron emission tomography (PET) has raised new possibilities for defining disease activity and monitoring response to therapy.[95] However, few centres have access to this technique and it has no role in routine clinical practice yet.

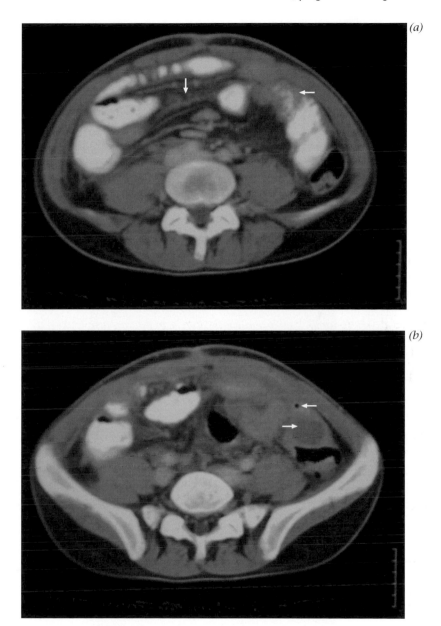

(a)

(b)

Figure 2.11 *Crohn's collection seen on CT scan. CT after oral and intravenous contrast medium administration. In the more craniad image (a) thickening of the small bowel is seen (←) with stranding within the mesentery (↓). In the lower image (b) a fluid collection with a thick wall (→) is seen just posterior to another, adherent thickened loop of bowel (←). (Reproduced courtesy of Dr J Hughes, Guy's Hospital, London.)*

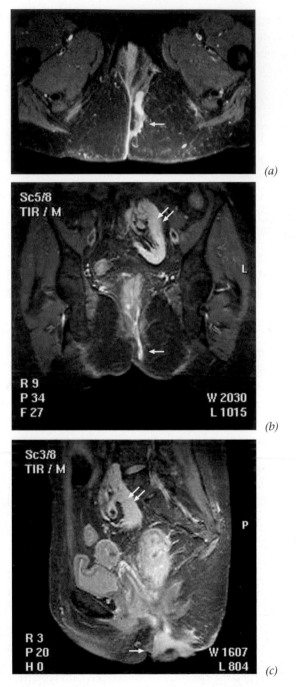

Figure 2.12 *Magnetic resonance imaging appearances of perianal fistula in Crohn's disease. Axial (a), coronal (b), and sagittal (c) MR images (STIR sequence) of a perianal fistula (←) seen in all three imaging planes. (There is a renal transplant in the left iliac fossa (↙)). (Reproduced courtesy of Dr G Rottenberg, Guy's Hospital, London.)*

Conclusions

The various imaging techniques outlined above have complementary roles in the diagnosis and management of Crohn's disease (Table 2.6). How they should be selected in making a diagnosis of Crohn's disease and in managing its different presentations is outlined below and in Chapter 6.

Assessment of activity of Crohn's disease

In ordinary clinical practice, as indicated above, disease activity is usually assessed on the basis of the patient's symptoms and signs, together with simple blood tests. Ileocolonoscopy and/or radiolabelled leukocyte scans may also be helpful in equivocal cases, for example patients with symptoms suggestive of relapse but without abnormal blood test results.

Disease activity can be more formally quantified, mainly in the context of clinical trials, using a range of clinical and laboratory scores (Chapter 3).[76,96] The Crohn's disease activity index (CDAI) is the most widely used and is calculated from a prospective seven-day symptom diary, abdominal examination, the presence of extraintestinal manifestations, weight and haematocrit (Table 2.7).[97] Scores above 150 are taken to indicate active Crohn's, 151 to 400 mild-moderate disease and over 450, very severe disease.[97] The Harvey–Bradshaw index is calculated from a single assessment of symptoms, the presence or absence of an abdominal mass and complications; it correlates well with CDAI and is easier to calculate (Table 2.8).[98] The limitations of such scoring systems are described in Chapter 3.

Table 2.6 Usefulness of imaging techniques for assessment of Crohn's disease.[100]

	Site	*Activity*	*Complications**
Conventional radiology			
Plain abdominal film	+	+	−
Barium follow-through	+ +	+ +	+
Ileocolonoscopy and biopsy	+ +	+ +	+
Newer imaging techniques			
Radiolabelled leukocyte scan	+	+ +	+
Ultrasound	+	+	+
Computed tomography	+	+	+ +
Magnetic resonance imaging	+	+	+ +

*Abscess, fistula, perianal disease.

Table 2.7 Crohn's disease activity index.[97]

Variable	Points given	Subtotal
Number of liquid or very soft stools each day for 1 week	Total number added together for week	Multiply number × 2
Abdominal pain rating each day for 1 week	0 = none 1 = mild 2 = moderate 3 = severe Add together each day's total	Multiply number × 5
General well-being each day for one week	0 = generally well 1 = slightly under par 2 = poor 3 = very poor 4 = terrible Add together total for each day	Multiply number × 7
Number of six listed categories that patient now has	(a) arthritis/athralgia (b) iritis/uveitis (c) erythema nodosum/ pyoderma gangrenosum/ aphthous stomatitis (d) anal fissure/fistula/abscess (e) other fistula (f) fever over 100 °F (37.8 °C) in last week Add together number	Multiply number × 20
Taking loperamide or opiates to control diarrhoea	0 = no 1 = yes	Multiply number × 30
Presence of abdominal mass	0 = none 2 = questionable 5 = definite	Multiply number × 10
Haematocrit	Male = 47 minus haematocrit Female = 42 minus haematocrit	Multiply number × 6
Current body weight	Percentage difference between this and standard weight	Multiply figure × 1 Then either add this figure (underweight) or subtract it (overweight)
	Total	**CDAI = ___ points**

Table 2.8 Harvey–Bradshaw index of Crohn's disease activity.[98]

Variable	Points given
General well-being	0 = very well 1 = slightly below par 2 = poor 3 = very poor 4 = terrible
Abdominal pain	0 = none 1 = mild 2 = moderate 3 = severe
Number of liquid stools per day	Total
Abdominal mass	0 = none 1 = dubious 2 = definite 3 = definite and tender
Complications: arthralgia, uveitis, erythema nodosum, aphthous ulcers, pyoderma gangrenosum, anal fissure, new fistula, abscess	Score 1 for each item
Total	**Harvey–Bradshaw index** ___

Differential diagnosis of Crohn's disease

The differential diagnoses of common presentations of Crohn's disease are shown in Tables 2.9–2.13 and suggested approaches to investigation in Figures 2.13–2.15. In younger patients (under 50 years), the most common differential diagnoses, depending on presentation, include infection and irritable bowel syndrome. In older people, neoplasia, diverticular disease and ischaemia require special consideration. In each case a careful history and examination will elicit the features which may point to a particular route and selection of investigations. Rarely, there are no clues to aetiology and in these cases a methodical approach should lead to the diagnosis.

Table 2.9 Causes of bloody diarrhoea.[99]

Inflammatory	Ulcerative colitis
	Crohn's disease
	Behçet's disease
Infective colitis	Campylobacter
	Shigella
	Salmonella
	Clostridium difficile
	Yersinia
	Tuberculosis
	Enterohaemorrhagic *Escherichia coli* (VTEC/0157:H7)
	Amoebiasis
	Schistosomiasis
	Cytomegalovirus*
	Herpes simplex virus*
Neoplastic	Colorectal carcinoma
Vascular	Ischaemia
Iatrogenic	NSAIDs
	Antibiotics
	Irradiation

*Particularly in immunocompromised patients.
VTEC, verocytotoxin-producing *E. coli* serotype 0157:H7; NSAIDs, non-steroidal anti-inflammatory drugs.

Table 2.10 Causes of rectal bleeding.[99]

Inflammatory	Ulcerative colitis
	Crohn's disease
Anal disease	Haemorrhoids
	Fissure
Sexually transmitted	Gonococcus
	Cytomegalovirus
	Herpes simplex virus
	Atypical mycobacterium
	Chlamydia
	Kaposi's sarcoma
Neoplasia	Colorectal polyps
	Colorectal carcinoma
	Anal cancer
Vascular	Ischaemia
	Angiodysplasia
Iatrogenic	NSAIDs (oral or suppositories)
	Irradiation
Other	Benign solitary rectal ulcer
	Diverticulosis (acute bleed only)
	Severe upper GI haemorrhage

NSAIDs, non-steroidal anti-inflammatory drugs.

Table 2.11 Causes of diarrhoea, abdominal pain and weight loss.[99]

Inflammatory	Crohn's disease
	Ulcerative colitis
	Microscopic/collagenous/lymphocytic colitis*
	Behçet's disease
Neoplasia	Colorectal carcinoma
	Pancreatic cancer
	Small bowel lymphoma
	Endocrine tumours (e.g. VIPoma, carcinoid)
Endocrine	Thyrotoxicosis
	Diabetic autonomic neuropathy
	Hypoadrenalism
Vascular	Ischaemia
Infection	See Table 2.9
Iatrogenic	NSAIDs
	Antibiotics
	Laxative abuse
	Irradiation
	Gut resections
Malabsorption	Coeliac disease
	Bacterial overgrowth
	Lactose intolerance†
Other	Irritable bowel syndrome†

*Pain and weight loss unusual.
†Weight loss unusual.
VIP, vasoactive intestinal polypeptide; NSAIDs, non-steroidal anti-inflammatory drugs.

Table 2.12 Causes of abdominal pain and mass in the right iliac fossa.[99]

Ileocaecal	Inflammatory	Crohn's disease
		Appendix mass
	Infective	Tuberculosis
		Amoeboma
		Actinomycosis
	Neoplastic	Caecal carcinoma
		Lymphoma
		Carcinoid tumour
	Other	Faecal loading
Renal	Hydronephrosis	
	Cysts	
	Neoplasia	
	Transplant	
Gynaecological	Ovarian cyst	
	Neoplasia	
	Tubal mass, including ectopic pregnancy	
	Endometriosis	

Table 2.13 Differential diagnosis of perianal ulceration.[101]

Inflammatory	Crohn's disease
	Behçet's syndrome
Infection	Herpes simplex
	Syphilis
	Tuberculosis
	Lymphogranuloma venereum
Neoplasia	Anal carcinoma

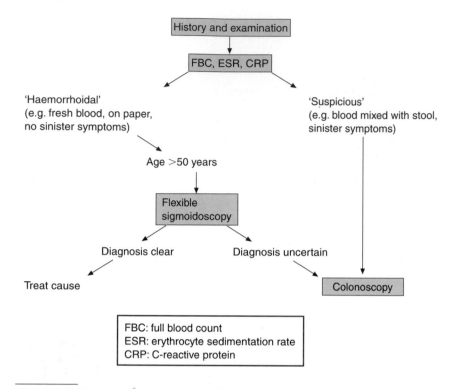

Figure 2.13 Investigation of chronic and minor rectal bleeding. (Adapted with permission from Lim. In: Rampton DS, ed. Inflammatory Bowel Disease, Clinical Diagnosis and Management. *London: Martin Dunitz, 2000, 71–85.*[101])

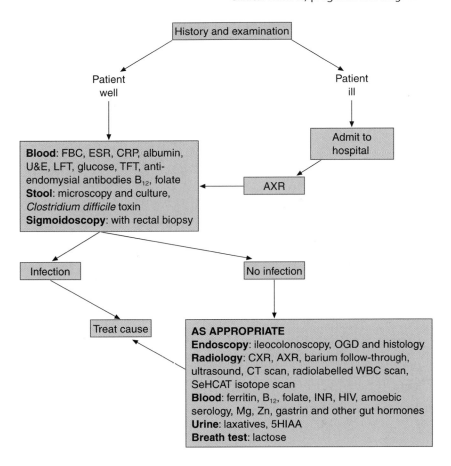

History and examination

Patient well

Patient ill

Admit to hospital

Blood: FBC, ESR, CRP, albumin, U&E, LFT, glucose, TFT, anti-endomysial antibodies B_{12}, folate
Stool: microscopy and culture, *Clostridium difficile* toxin
Sigmoidoscopy: with rectal biopsy

AXR

Infection

No infection

Treat cause

AS APPROPRIATE
Endoscopy: ileocolonoscopy, OGD and histology
Radiology: CXR, AXR, barium follow-through, ultrasound, CT scan, radiolabelled WBC scan, SeHCAT isotope scan
Blood: ferritin, B_{12}, folate, INR, HIV, amoebic serology, Mg, Zn, gastrin and other gut hormones
Urine: laxatives, 5HIAA
Breath test: lactose

FBC: full blood count
ESR: erythrocyte sedimentation rate
CRP: C-reactive protein
LFT: liver function tests
TFT: thyroid function tests
U&E: urea and electrolytes
CXR/AXR: chest/abdominal radiograph
OGD: oesophagogastroduodenoscopy
5HIAA: 5-hydroxyindoleacetic acid
SeHCAT: ^{75}Se-homocholic acid test
INR: International normalised ratio
HIV: human immunodeficiency virus
CT: computed tomography

Figure 2.14 *Investigation of diarrhoea (with or without blood).*

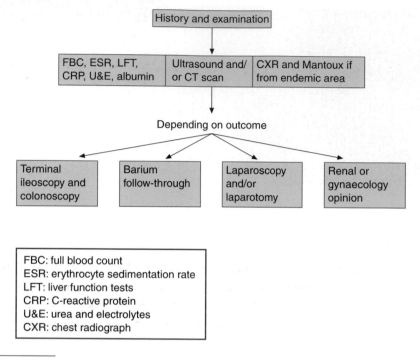

Figure 2.15 Investigation of mass in right iliac fossa.

chapter 3

Drug treatment of Crohn's disease

Introduction

This chapter describes current and future pharmacological options available for the specific and supportive treatment of the intestinal manifestations of Crohn's disease (Table 3.1). Additional therapy is described in Chapter 5. How the various current alternatives are used in clinical practice is covered in Chapters 6 and 9.

Investigating new therapies for IBD: principles

It is beyond the scope of this book to discuss the preclinical development of new therapies for IBD and in particular how their pharmacological effects are modelled and tested in man and animals.[46,102]

As in other areas of medicine, the key test of the therapeutic usefulness of a new agent for Crohn's is the randomized clinical trial: the design and interpretation of such trials in Crohn's are, however, unusually difficult, for reasons outlined below.

Clinical trials in IBD

Investigation of the clinical efficacy of new drugs in Crohn's disease is not straightforward. Confounding factors common to other diseases, such as mistaken diagnosis, comorbidity, poor compliance and inadequate dosage or duration of therapy, will not be considered further here. Instead, we review some of the problems of trial design, execution and interpretation which are particular to Crohn's.[103–105]

Table 3.1 Current evidence-based pharmacological options for the specific and supportive treatment of Crohn's disease.

Group	Example
Disease specific therapies	
Corticosteroids	Prednisolone
	Budesonide
Aminosalicylates (5-ASA)	Pentasa
	Asacol
	Sulphasalazine
Antibiotics	Metronidazole
	Ciprofloxacin
	Clarithromycin
Immunomodulators	Thiopurines (azathioprine/6-mercaptopurine)
	Methotrexate
	Mycophenolate mofetil
Anti-TNF agents	Infliximab
	Thalidomide
*Supportive therapies**	
Antidiarrhoeals	Loperamide
	Codeine phosphate
Bile salt binding agents	Cholestyramine
	Colestipol

*Other supportive drugs, such as haematinics, are discussed in Chapter 9.

Disease heterogeneity

Because of the waxing and waning natural history of Crohn's disease, clinical trials have to be aimed clearly either at induction of remission in patients with active disease or at remission maintenance in subjects with disease quiescent at recruitment.

In the latter setting, factors influencing the likelihood of relapse should be matched in the control and test patient groups. These include site of disease and its behaviour (penetrating or non-penetrating),[106] time since previous relapse or surgery and smoking habit.[22]

The inflammation in Crohn's affects a varying extent of the bowel, anywhere from mouth to anus (Chapter 2). This has important implications for the response to particular drug delivery systems. For example, oral formulations of aminosalicylates or budesonide in which the active agent is released in the distal ileum and proximal colon are unlikely to work in patients with proximal small intestinal disease or left-sided Crohn's colitis.

The symptoms of Crohn's disease may be due to a variety of different pathological processes, ranging from mucosal inflammation through stricturing to abscess and fistula formation (Chapter 2): patients with different pathological explanations for their presentation will show different responses to a particular therapy.

Other factors influencing response to a trial drug include concurrent therapy and the time since discontinuation of previous treatments: the effectiveness of thiopurines, for example, may take up to four months to abate. Influences less easy to identify in planning recruitment are changes in gut physiology which may alter a test drug's pharmacokinetics: these include malabsorption due to small intestinal disease and abnormalities of gut pH and transit.[107]

Certain genotypes provide a clue to disease behaviour and response to therapy (Chapter 1). For example, *NOD2* mutations are associated with fistulizing ileal and right colonic disease, stenosis and the need for resection.[14] Genotype may also determine response to drugs such as thiopurines, steroids, methotrexate, ciclosporin and infliximab.[108–110] Unrecognized genotypic differences between patients are likely to explain much of the variability of response in clinical trials.

Trial design

The heterogeneity of Crohn's means that clinical trials should be stratified prospectively to minimize differences between groups of patients treated with novel and comparator (or placebo) drugs. Unfortunately, however, most trials have been too small to match patient groups satisfactorily.

Argument persists as to whether a novel agent should be compared with an existing therapy or placebo. In severe disease, a placebo is clearly unethical. However, many clinicians feel that use of a placebo group in patients with mild-moderately active Crohn's allows the clearest initial assessment of a new agent. In placebo-controlled studies, the trial can usually be smaller than when standard comparator therapy is used, since the difference sought in power studies will be larger: this results in exposure of fewer subjects to the novel agent, an important consideration in relation to possible toxicity and failure of efficacy of new drugs. If placebos are used, prompt withdrawal of patients must occur if they fail to respond or deteriorate. Cognisance should be taken too of the size and variability of the placebo response in Crohn's.[57]

Objective measurement of disease activity and definition of outcome is particularly contentious in Crohn's disease.[103,111] There is a lack of hard end-points, death being too rare in Crohn's to be a useful measure of therapeutic efficacy. Outcome measures employed include clinical activity indices and quality of life scores, achievement of predetermined therapeutic goals, laboratory measures of inflammation and mucosal appearances, as well as adverse drug effects.

Clinical activity indices

There is a wide range of clinical activity indices for Crohn's disease (Chapter 2).[76,96] The multiplicity of such scores indicates their inadequacy. Difficulties include the unreliability of symptom recording by patients, inappropriate weighting of certain variables in some scoring systems, the poor correlation between clinical scores and disease activity assessed biochemically and endoscopically,[80] and the consequent difficulty in defining remission and/or clinically significant improvement. Despite these problems, activity indices such as the CDAI (Table 2.7)[97] and the simpler Harvey–Bradshaw index (Table 2.8)[98] are widely used to evaluate clinical activity in therapeutic trials in Crohn's.

Quality of life scores

There is increasing interest in quality of life scores to assess response in clinical trials in IBD.[112,113] To date, however, there is insufficient experience to suggest that such methods should be used as primary rather than secondary outcome measures in trials in Crohn's.[111]

Therapeutic goals

To obviate some of the problems associated with clinical scoring systems, specified goals have been proposed as outcome measures. These have included reduction of steroid dosage,[114] avoidance of surgery, fistula closure[115] and prevention of endoscopic recurrence after surgery.[82] Such goals have the advantage of being well-defined and of clinical relevance.

Laboratory measures of inflammation

Unfortunately, no single blood test or set of tests is a reliable measure of therapeutic response (Chapter 2).[76] Four-day faecal excretion of indium-labelled leukocytes may provide a better guide,[116] but is cumbersome for the patient and involves exposure to radio-isotopes. Whether measurement of faecal excretion of calprotectin[117] will fulfil its early promise remains to be seen.

Mucosal appearance and histology

The mucosal appearances at colonoscopy can be scored semi-objectively in Crohn's colitis[118] and at the ileo-colonic anastomosis after surgery.[82] Indeed, it has been proposed that the primary goal of therapy in Crohn's should be endoscopic mucosal healing.[119,120]

No score to assess inflammation microscopically in Crohn's has achieved widespread usage. Furthermore, the patchy distribution of inflammation in Crohn's disease may lead to a risk of sampling error.

Assessment of mucosal response to novel therapies requires repeated endoscopy, a procedure which is neither pleasant nor entirely safe. Furthermore, in patients with mid-small bowel Crohn's disease, the mucosa is inaccessible to endoscopic examination, at least until further experience with the wireless capsule endoscope has been gained.[83]

Conclusion

To address the problems outlined above, the clinical trials taskforce of the International Organization of Inflammatory Bowel Disease has published a consensus statement to try to reduce inconsistencies between trials.[111]

Standard drugs

Corticosteroids

Mechanisms of action

Both classes of the effects of corticosteroids, mineralocorticoid and glucocorticoid, are determined by their binding to intracellular receptors (Figure 3.1).[121] Mineralocorticoid effects are mediated through type I receptors and promote renal and colonic retention of sodium and water and loss of potassium. Glucocorticoid receptors (type II) affect the synthesis of inflammatory mediators, neutrophil function and cellular immunity[121] (Table 3.2). For treating inflammatory diseases such as Crohn's, the aim is to use a potent glucocorticoid with minimal mineralocorticoid activity.

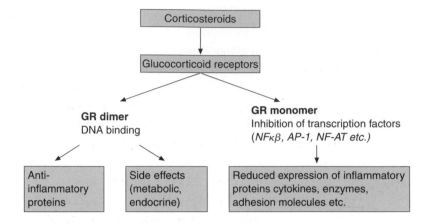

Figure 3.1 *Receptor types and pharmacological effects of corticosteroids. GR, glucocorticoid receptors; NFκβ, nuclear factor κβ; AP-1, activator protein-1; NF-AT, nuclear factor of activated T cells. (Reproduced from Barnes.* Nature *1999; **402**: B31–8.[121])*

Table 3.2 Mechanisms of action of glucocorticoids.[312]

Cell type	Action
Leukocytes	Reduced migration, activation, survival
	Reduced activation of NFκβ
	Reduced production of proinflammatory cytokines
	(IL-1, -2, -6, -8, TNF-α)
	Phospholipase A2 inhibition
	Reduced induction of COX-2 and iNOS
	Reduced production of leukotrienes, thromboxanes,
	prostaglandins, PAF
	Increased kinin degradation
Endothelial cells	Reduced expression of adhesion molecules
	Reduced capillary permeability

NFκβ, nuclear transcription factor κβ; COX-2, cyclooxygenase-2; iNOS, inducible nitric oxide synthase; PAF, platelet activating factor.

Preparations

Corticosteroids are given orally, topically (rectal) or intravenously. Prednisolone is the most commonly used oral preparation. There is no good evidence that an enteric-coated preparation (Prednisolone EC) reduces dyspeptic symptoms. Prednisone, which is converted in the liver to prednisolone, has no special advantages.

The usual starting dose of prednisolone in active Crohn's is 40–60 mg daily until symptoms resolve (usually 7–28 days). Thereafter, the dose is tapered by 5 mg/day every 7–10 days.[122] Hydrocortisone (300–400 mg/day in divided doses) and methylprednisolone (40–60 mg/day in divided doses) are the two medications most commonly given intravenously for patients with very severe disease or who are unable to take an oral preparation.[122]

Budesonide is a potent glucocorticoid, which is given orally in a controlled-release preparation (Budenofalk, Entocort CR) to act specifically on the ileo-caecal region. Its rapid intestinal and hepatic first-pass metabolism reduces unwanted side-effects and results in less adrenocortical suppression than prednisolone.[123,124] The efficacy of budesonide in treating active ileocaecal Crohn's disease using a dose of 9 mg once daily exceeds that of Pentasa (an aminosalicylate) 4 g/day,[125] but does not quite reach that of prednisolone 40 mg/day.[124,126] Efforts are underway to develop preparations that release budesonide (as well as prednisolone) in the colon for patients with colitis.

For left-sided colonic, rectal and anal disease, topically applied cortico-steroids can be used. Topical therapy rarely causes systemic side-effects, but these can be further minimized using corticosteroids with rapid first-pass metabolism. These include prednisolone metasulphobenzoate (Predenema, Predfoam enema) and budesonide (Entocort enemas).

Indications

The primary indication for the use of corticosteroids is active disease. There is scant evidence that corticosteroids are of benefit in maintaining remission.[122,127,128]

Approximately 65% of patients with active Crohn's given prednisolone at 40–60 mg/day enter remission over three to four months, compared with 30% of those receiving placebo;[127,129] it is possible that failure of steroid responsiveness is associated with excessive expression of the multi-drug resistance (MDR) gene.[130] Controlled ileal release budesonide (9 mg/day) induces remission in 50–60% of patients with active ileocaecal Crohn's.[123,124]

In maintenance studies, budesonide 6 mg/day prolonged the time to relapse compared with 3 mg/day or placebo, but at one year did not improve remission rates (about 40%).[131,132] Despite the low risk of side-effects with long-term budesonide 6 mg/day, it is hard to justify its use for maintenance therapy except in patients in whom even a minor prolongation of remission is essential.

Side-effects
Unwanted corticosteroid side-effects are summarized in Table 3.3; most are dose- and duration-related.

Contra-indications
Poorly controlled diabetes mellitus, hypertension, peptic ulceration and osteoporosis may be worsened during treatment with corticosteroids. In patients with these problems who have ileocaecal Crohn's and in whom corticosteroid use is unavoidable, budesonide is preferable to prednisolone.

Monitoring treatment
In patients on high-dose corticosteroids, blood pressure, serum glucose and potassium levels should be monitored. For patients needing more than short courses of prednisolone, and particularly those who have taken a cumulative dose exceeding 10 g of prednisolone, bone densitometry (DEXA scanning) and treatment to prevent and treat osteoporosis are given[133] (Chapter 9, Figure 9.7).

Conclusions
While about 65% of patients given prednisolone achieve remission or improve symptomatically, at least half will relapse or become steroid-dependent one year after starting treatment.[2,134,135] Factors predisposing to steroid resistance and/or steroid dependency, defined as an inability to wean the patient off the drug without a return of symptoms, include younger age at diagnosis, a high CDAI, smoking, previous bowel resections, colonic and anoperineal disease.[136]

Table 3.3 Side effects of corticosteroids.[312]

Organ or system	Side-effect
Skin	Acne, purpura, moon-face, hirsuties, striae
Metabolic	Hyperglycaemia, hypokalaemia, adrenocortical suppression
Musculoskeletal	Osteoporosis, avascular osteonecrosis, growth retardation in children, myopathy
Cardiovascular	Hypertension, fluid retention
Infection	Opportunistic infection, reactivation of tuberculosis, severe chickenpox
Eyes	Cataract, glaucoma
Other	Weight gain, dysphoria, dyspepsia

More fundamentally, while corticosteroids reduce symptoms of active Crohn's in most patients, they improve colonoscopic appearances in only about 10% of patients: there is a poor correlation between the response to steroids as assessed by CDAI and by endoscopic severity index (CDEIS).[80,118] These findings suggest that steroids do little to down-regulate mucosal inflammation and are unlikely to improve the natural history of Crohn's disease.

The role of steroids should therefore be considered as principally ameliorative.[135] Their use should be restricted in dose and duration, so as to minimize side-effects (Table 3.3). Wherever possible, safer alternative therapies such as aminosalicylates and antibiotics should be used as first-line therapy in mild-moderately active disease. Furthermore, thiopurines or surgery should be considered early in patients showing evidence of dependency or side-effects on corticosteroids, to allow their withdrawal.

Aminosalicylates (5-ASA)

Mechanisms of action
Aminosalicylates have many anti-inflammatory effects (Table 3.4), but the mechanism of their efficacy in Crohn's is unknown.[137,138]

Table 3.4 Possible mechanisms of action of 5-ASA drugs.[312]

Immune system	Mechanism
Leukocytes	Reduced migration, cytotoxicity
	Reduced activation of NF$\kappa\beta$
	Reduced IL-1 and IL-12 synthesis
	Reduced synthesis of leukotrienes, thromboxanes, prostaglandins, PAF
	Reduced degradation of prostaglandins
	Antioxidant
	Reduced inducible nitric oxide synthase expression
	TNF-α antagonist
	Blocks formyl-methionyl-leucyl-phenylalanine (FMLP) receptors
Epithelium	Reduced MHC class II expression
	Induction of heat shock proteins
	Reduced apoptosis

PAF, platelet activating factor; NF$\kappa\beta$, nuclear transcription factor $\kappa\beta$; TNF-α, tumour necrosis factor-α; IL, interleukin.

Preparations

Available preparations are listed in Table 3.5, although formal evidence for efficacy in Crohn's exists only for Pentasa, Asacol and sulphasalazine.

The topically active component of the aminosalicylates, 5-ASA, is absorbed proximally in the bowel unless specially formulated. There are now several oral preparations which release 5-ASA distally in inflamed areas of the gut. The first was sulphasalazine, consisting of a sulphonamide carrier (sulphapyridine) linked by an azo bond to a 5-ASA molecule (Figure 3.2). The sulphonamide moiety carries the active compound to the colon where it is released by bacterial cleavage of the azo bond. Most of the side-effects associated with sulphasalazine (shown in Table 3.6) result from the sulphonamide carrier.

Olsalazine, which is made up of two 5-ASA compounds linked by azo bonds, and balsalazide, in which 5-ASA is azo bonded to aminobenzoylalanine (Figure 3.2), act only in the colon (Figure 3.3); these agents are of proven efficacy in UC but not yet in Crohn's colitis. Asacol and Salofalk are pH-dependent delayed-release preparations which deliver 5-ASA primarily to the ileocaecal region when the intraluminal pH exceeds 6–7 (Table 3.5). Pentasa, in contrast, starts to release 5-ASA more proximally in the small bowel from ethylcellulose microspheres (Table 3.5).

Table 3.5 Oral formulations: 5-aminosalicylate drugs.[312]

Drug	Formulation	Delivery site	Dose
Prodrugs (5-ASA linked to carrier)			
Sulphasalazine	5-ASA-sulphapyridine	Colon	1 g bd to 2 g tds
Olsalazine	5-ASA-5-ASA	Colon	500 mg bd to 1 g tds
Balsalazide	5-ASA-aminobenzoylalanine	Colon	1.5 g bd to 2.25 g tds
Mesalazine (5-ASA alone)			
Delayed release			
Asacol	Eudragit S coating dissolving at pH >7	Distal ileum, colon	400 mg tds to 1.2 g tds
Salofalk	Eudragit L coating dissolving at pH >6	Ileum, colon	500 mg tds to 1 g tds
Slow-release			
Pentasa	Ethylcellulose microspheres	Duodenum to colon	500 mg tds to 2 g bd

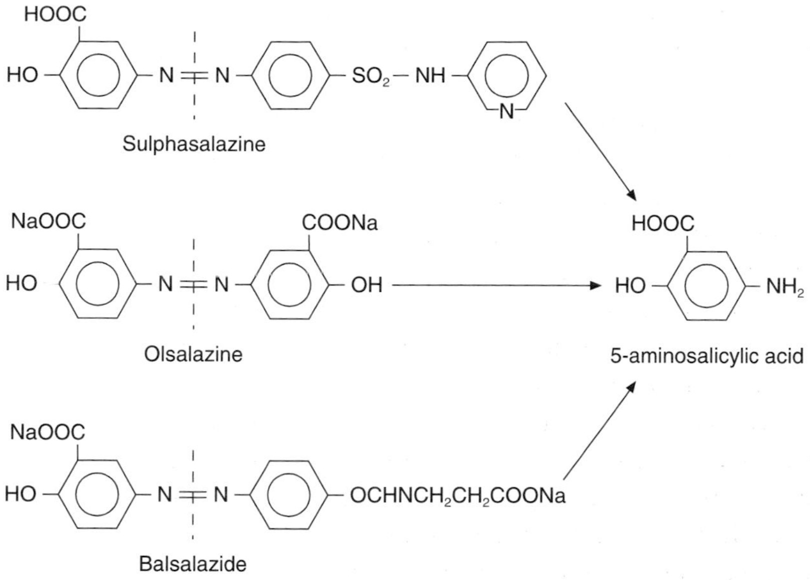

Figure 3.2 *Chemical formulations of 5-aminosalicylates.*

Table 3.6 Side-effects of 5-ASA drugs.[312]

System or organ	Side-effect
General	Headache,* fever*
Gut	Nausea,* vomiting,* diarrhoea
Blood	Haemolysis,* folate deficiency,* agranulocytosis,* thrombocytopaenia,* aplastic anaemia,* methaemoglobinaemia*
Skin	Rashes,* toxic necrolysis,* Stevens-Johnson syndrome,* hair loss
Renal	Orange urine,* interstitial nephritis
Other	Oligospermia,* acute pancreatitis, hepatitis, lupus syndrome, myocarditis, pulmonary fibrosis
Drug interactions	Leukopenia in patients on thiopurines

*Denotes side-effects usually but not always associated with the sulphonamide component of sulphasalazine.

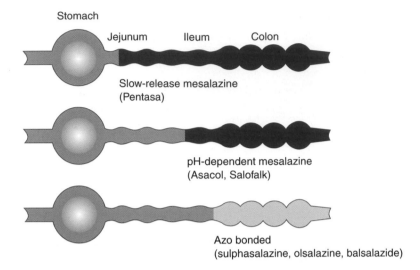

Stomach
Jejunum   Ileum   Colon

Slow-release mesalazine
(Pentasa)

pH-dependent mesalazine
(Asacol, Salofalk)

Azo bonded
(sulphasalazine, olsalazine, balsalazide)

Figure 3.3 *Diagram of sites where 5-aminosalicylate preparations are released (Reproduced with permission from Rampton and Shanahan.* Fast Facts – Inflammatory Bowel Disease. *Oxford: Health Press, 2000.[99])*

There is no evidence about the efficacy of 5-ASA liquid enemas, foams or suppositories in distal colorectal Crohn's disease, despite their proven value in UC.

Indications

Aminosalicylates, in high dose, have some benefit in patients with mild-moderately active Crohn's disease. Sulphasalazine 4–6 g/day is superior to placebo in Crohn's colitis,[127] but is not well tolerated. Pentasa and Asacol in doses above 3.2 g/day also induce remission in mild-moderately active Crohn's;[139–141] however, the former was less effective than budesonide 9 mg/day.[125] Lower doses of 5-ASA preparations have no effect in active Crohn's.

Meta-analysis shows that aminosalicylates are ineffective in maintaining remission in patients with medically induced remissions.[142] They may have some efficacy in patients with surgically induced remissions, when disease is restricted to the small bowel[142–145] (Chapter 6).

Side-effects

Although better tolerated than sulphasalazine, the newer preparations also have some side-effects (Table 3.6). These vary from minor rashes, headache and nausea, through diarrhoea to pancreatitis and blood dyscrasias in up to

5% of patients. Bone marrow suppression can occur and the Committee on Safety of Medicines has recommended that all patients taking 5-ASA drugs report any bleeding, bruising, sore throats, fever or malaise.[146] Interstitial nephritis occurs in one in 500 patients.[147]

In patients taking azathioprine or 6-mercaptopurine, co-administration of mesalazine or sulphasalazine increases blood 6-thioguanine nucleotide concentrations by inhibition of the thiopurine-metabolizing enzyme, TPMT (see p. 58) and may increase the risk of leukopenia.[148,149]

Contra-indications

Aminosalicylates should be avoided in patients hypersensitive to salicylates, including aspirin, or with renal impairment. Sulphasalazine should be avoided in those with hypersensitivity to sulphonamides, porphyria or glucose-6-phosphate dehydrogenase deficiency.

Monitoring treatment

Patients on aminosalicylates should have a full blood count and checks of their urea and creatinine concentrations and liver function tests every 6–12 months.

Conclusions

In moderately high doses (about 4 g/day) aminosalicylates induce remission in 40–50% of patients with mildly active Crohn's, but it is not known whether still higher doses are safe and/or more efficacious. As indicated, the evidence for aminosalicylates as maintenance therapy is equivocal. Further studies are needed to confirm that Pentasa started early after surgery might be effective prophylaxis in patients with exclusively small bowel disease.[143] It remains to be seen whether combinations of 5-ASA with, for example, a thiopurine (see below) might have a beneficial effect postoperatively.

Antibiotics

Metronidazole

Mechanism of action. As a nitroimidazole antibiotic, metronidazole may act by reducing the mucosal immunological reaction initiated and sustained by anaerobic luminal bacteria (Chapter 1). It also has immunomodulatory and anti-inflammatory effects in vitro.[150]

Preparations. Although metronidazole can be given intravenously and rectally, the only data relating to Crohn's concern the oral tablet.

Indications. In a comparison of sulphasalazine and metronidazole for active Crohn's disease, there was no difference between the two drugs; however, only 25% of patients responded and low doses of metronidazole were used (400 mg bd).[151] In a placebo-controlled study, metronidazole (10–20 mg/kg per day) increased the probability of obtaining but not maintaining remission and worked in colonic rather than ileal disease.[152] Another study showed no increase in remission rate with short-term metronidazole given singly or with co-trimoxazole over placebo.[153] The effects of metronidazole may be enhanced by co-administration of ciprofloxacin in ileocolonic and colonic disease,[154,155] but adequate controlled data are lacking. The role of metronidazole in perianal Crohn's disease[156] will be discussed in Chapter 6. Lastly, a placebo-controlled trial of patients with ileal Crohn's disease entering surgically induced remission showed that metronidazole at 20 mg/kg per day for three months reduced clinical recurrence at one year but not thereafter.[157]

Side-effects and contra-indications. Side-effects range from rashes, nausea, vomiting, an unpleasant taste in the mouth and an 'Antabuse' effect after alcohol to serious sensory peripheral neuropathy, which may be irreversible and limits the duration of treatment to three months.[158]

Other antibiotics. Limited data suggest that ciprofloxacin alone[159,160] or with metronidazole[154,155] may have a role in mild-moderately active Crohn's when given for up to six months. Uncontrolled reports also suggest therapeutic benefits for clarithromycin, rifabutin and clofazimine, singly or together,[30] although it is not certain that this effect is due to eradication of *Mycobacterium paratuberculosis* (Chapter 1). Conventional antituberculous triple therapy has not proved beneficial in Crohn's disease.[161] Antibiotics such as amoxicillin and metronidazole are useful for treating diarrhoea due to bacterial overgrowth in patients with small bowel Crohn's disease.

Immunomodulatory drugs

Azathioprine and 6-mercaptopurine

Mechanism of action and pharmacology. Azathioprine is a prodrug which is converted to 6-mercaptopurine (6MP) in the liver by glutathione transferase. 6MP is metabolized in the liver and gut by three main enzymes to 6-thioguanine nucleotides (6-TGN) (Figure 3.4), the compounds thought to be therapeutically active and to cause leukopenia and/or pancytopenia.

Homozygous and heterozygous deficiencies of TPMT (thiopurine methyl-transferase) occur in about 0.2 and 10% of the population respectively and they predispose to the serious side-effects, particularly bone marrow suppression, occasionally encountered with thiopurines.[162–164] Conversely, low TPMT levels, by causing an increase in intracellular 6-TGN in lymphocytes, may improve the clinical efficacy of the thiopurines. Assays of TPMT genotype or activity, and of erythrocyte 6-TGN levels, are not yet widely available routinely, nor is it yet clear how measurement of these variables will help dose selection.[164] The only exception to this uncertainty at present is that, if TPMT genotype or activity can be measured and the patient is found to be

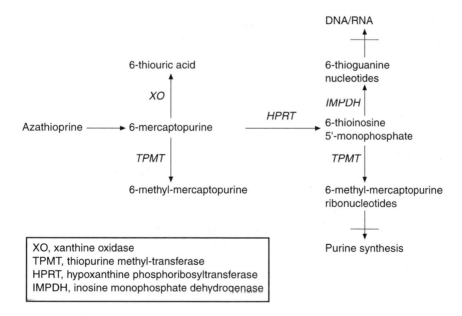

Figure 3.4 Breakdown of thiopurine drugs. (Reproduced from Dubinsky et al. Gastroenterology 2000; **118**: 705–13 with permission from American Gastroenterological Association.)

homozygous for its deficiency, thiopurines should be avoided altogether. Note, however, that serious toxicity to both azathioprine and 6-MP may be seen even in the presence of normal TPMT levels.[163]

The thiopurines appear to inhibit T- and B-lymphocyte proliferation as a result of the gradual intracellular accumulation of 6-TGNs and their inhibition of RNA and DNA synthesis.[163] There is evidence that azathioprine may also have an antibiotic effect against anaerobes.[165]

Preparations. Azathioprine and 6-MP are given orally at doses of 2–2.5 mg/kg per day and 1–1.5 mg/kg per day, respectively, and take up to 16 weeks to work. There is no evidence that intravenous azathioprine can reduce this delay despite the rapid achievement of high erythrocyte concentrations of 6-TGNs.[166]

Indications. Although they are not licensed for this indication in the UK, there is strong evidence that the thiopurines are effective steroid-sparing agents in steroid-dependent and steroid-refractory Crohn's.[167–169] Meta-analysis from 8 placebo-controlled trials has shown that 56% of patients with active disease given thiopurines had a clinical response in four months, compared with 32% of patients on placebo; there was concomitant steroid-sparing.[168,169] Combinations of either azathioprine or 6-MP with prednisolone may heal refractory ileal and fistulating perianal disease.[119,168] By achieving mucosal healing, it is conceivable that azathioprine could improve the natural history of Crohn's.[119]

The remission-maintaining and steroid-sparing actions of the thiopurines suggest that they should be used long term. However, their consequent therapeutic benefits need to be counterbalanced against potential toxicity (see below). Controlled data suggest that in patients successfully maintained in remission on a thiopurine, the risk of relapse after four years of treatment is similar whether the drug is continued or stopped.[170]

Side-effects. Approximately 20% of patients given azathioprine develop nausea, upper abdominal discomfort, headache, rash, fever and/or arthralgia soon after starting the drug (Table 3.7). Some of these symptoms may be due to the imidazole group of azathioprine.[171] In about 50% of affected patients, a change to 6-MP may avert these non-specific side-effects and allow continued thiopurine therapy.[172,173]

More serious problems include acute pancreatitis, which occurs in about 3% of patients, usually in the first few weeks of treatment, and cholestatic hepatitis

Table 3.7 Side-effects of thiopurines.[312]

Organ or system	Side-effect
General	Nausea, vomiting, headache, arthralgia, fever, rash, abdominal pain
Blood	Agranulocytosis, thrombocytopenia, macrocytosis
Hepatobiliary	Acute pancreatitis, cholestatic hepatitis
Infections	Cytomegalovirus, herpes zoster, Epstein–Barr virus
Malignancy	Lymphoma (possibly), skin

(0.3%). Bone marrow suppression is often but not always associated with TPMT deficiency,[164] other contributory causes including Epstein–Barr virus infection and 5'nucleotidase deficiency. This side-effect occurs in about 2% of patients, again usually during the first weeks of therapy, and necessitates strict monitoring with blood tests (see below). There is an increased risk of opportunistic infections including cytomegalovirus, herpes zoster and Epstein–Barr virus.[174]

Any increased risk of lymphoma in patients given thiopurines for IBD appears to be minimal.[75] This risk seems to be lower than for patients immunosuppressed after kidney or liver transplantation,[175] but may be associated particularly with Epstein–Barr virus infection.[176] Thiopurines increase the risk of skin cancer[177] and fair-skinned patients should be warned to avoid sunbathing. The risk of other cancers after azathioprine does not seem to be increased in IBD.[178]

In a systematic review of maintenance azathioprine, the withdrawal rate for adverse effects was 6% in long-term follow-up.[169]

Contra-indications. Where TPMT assays prior to therapy are available, identification of homozygous deficiency means that thiopurines should not be used (see above). In heterozygotes, it may be possible to use low doses (e.g. azathioprine 1 mg/kg/day) so long as blood counts are very rigorously checked.

Allopurinol inhibits xanthine oxidase (see Figure 3.4). While use of allopurinol usually contra-indicates use of thiopurines, if monitoring of 6-TGN levels is available it may be possible to prescribe low doses of azathioprine or 6-MP safely (for example, 25 mg on alternate days) in patients needing allopurinol.

5-ASA drugs may raise red cell 6-TGN levels[149] by inhibiting 6-TPMT,[148] and thereby increase the risk of leukopenia. This does not appear to be a major clinical problem, but reinforces the need for regular monitoring of blood count.

Although azathioprine and 6-MP are theoretically teratogenic, small retrospective studies in which patients taking them have become pregnant have not shown any harm to the fetus.[179,180] There are limited data to suggest that women who conceive a child to a man taking a thiopurine are at increased risk of spontaneous abortion and congenital abnormalities in their baby,[181,182] but these drugs do not appear to affect male fertility.[179,183]

Monitoring treatment. Routine monitoring of patients on thiopurines should include full blood count every two weeks for the first two months of treatment to check for bone marrow depression. Thereafter, blood count and liver function tests every two months are advised.[184]

As indicated, the potential usefulness of measuring erythrocyte 6-TGN levels to monitor treatment efficacy and/or side-effects is not yet clear. For example, in clinical non-responders who have low 6-TGN levels, the dose of thiopurine might be increased to achieve higher, but non-toxic 6-TGN levels.[185] Such an approach may be useful in patients with high TPMT levels and consequently poor response to standard doses of thiopurines.

In relation to non-response, furthermore, it is not yet clear whether attempting to induce neutropenia by increasing the dose of azathioprine or 6-MP is either effective or safe.[186] Conversely, confirmation is needed that early development of macrocytosis after initiation of thiopurine therapy predicts a good clinical response.[187]

There are, as yet, no accepted guidelines about monitoring for the possible risk of lymphoma or other neoplasia in patients on long-term thiopurines; clearly, a low index of suspicion is required in patients deteriorating clinically during this treatment.

Conclusions. There are several outstanding questions limiting optimal use of thiopurines in Crohn's disease.

First, we need to define the value or otherwise of determining TPMT genotype or activity and 6-TGN levels. Indeed, further studies are needed to clarify the possible role and/or safety of oral 6-TG itself as treatment for Crohn's, particularly in TPMT-deficient patients.[188]

Second, the indications for use of thiopurines need to be further explored.

For example, further evaluation is needed of the possibility that they might reduce recurrence postoperatively (Chapter 6).[189,190] Early data suggest that thiopurines may reduce both the formation of antibodies to infliximab (ATI) and serum sickness-like reactions in patients given infliximab (see below).[191]

Further data are needed about the long-term safety of azathioprine and 6-MP, particularly in relation to neoplasia. We need to learn about how best to deal with thiopurine-induced leukopenia or abnormalities of liver function: it is not clear whether the drug should be discontinued altogether or its dosage merely reduced.

Lastly, a new colonic release preparation of azathioprine is under development;[192] whether this will be as efficacious as and/or safer than existing formulations for patients with Crohn's colitis remains to be seen.

Methotrexate

Mechanism of action. Methotrexate acts predominantly by inhibiting enzymes metabolizing folic acid. At high doses, the main enzyme affected is dihydrofolate reductase, with consequent inhibition of RNA, DNA and protein synthesis.[193,194] At the lower doses used to treat Crohn's disease, the anti-inflammatory and immunomodulatory effects of methotrexate are likely to result from inhibition of other folate-dependent enzymes.[194]

Preparations. Methotrexate is available in oral, intramuscular and subcutaneous preparations.

Indications. The largest trial in active Crohn's disease showed that methotrexate 25 mg/week given intramuscularly, at the same time as a tapering course of oral prednisolone, significantly increased the likelihood of obtaining remission (39%) over placebo (19%).[195] However, smaller studies have given equivocal or negative results, particularly with lower or oral doses of methotrexate.[196–198] Furthermore, side-effects (see below) led to drug withdrawal in 5–20% of patients. The time to remission was 16–24 weeks, resembling that of thiopurines.[195]

Methotrexate as maintenance therapy has been compared with placebo in patients achieving remission on intramuscular methotrexate.[195,199] Methotrexate, (15 mg/week) intramuscularly for 40 weeks, sustained remission in 65% of patients compared with 39% of those on placebo, and halved the use of prednisolone.[199] Oral preparations used in smaller trials showed a trend towards maintaining remission at 20 mg/week but not at 12.5 mg/week.[196,197]

Side-effects. Side-effects necessitate discontinuation of methotrexate in up to 20% of patients: nausea, vomiting, stomatitis and diarrhoea are the most common (Table 3.8).[197] As with other immunosuppressive agents, there is an increase in opportunistic infections. Bone marrow depression is common, occurring in 20% of patients receiving methotrexate for rheumatoid arthritis, and is usually reversible on stopping therapy or with dose reduction. All these side-effects are reduced by co-administration of folic acid, which does not compromise the therapeutic efficacy of methotrexate.[193,200]

Hepatic fibrosis and pneumonitis have been the most serious side-effects of long-term therapy with methotrexate in patients with psoriasis and rheumatoid arthritis.[201] A study of the hepatic effects of methotrexate in patients with IBD used liver biopsy at a cumulative dose of 1.5–5.4 g given over one to five years to grade hepatotoxicity.[202] Histological examination revealed that only one in 20 patients had developed liver fibrosis in the

Table 3.8 Side-effects of and contra-indications to methotrexate.

Side-effects

General	Nausea, vomiting, stomatitis, diarrhoea
Blood	Bone marrow depression
Hepatobiliary	Hepatic fibrosis
Infections	Opportunistic including *Pneumocystis carinii* pneumonia, Epstein–Barr virus, herpes zoster infections
Respiratory	Hypersensitivity pneumonitis
Malignancy	Lymphoproliferative disorders

Contra-indications

Pregnancy and childbirth Breast feeding	Avoid conception within 6 months for either partner
Drug interactions	Trimethoprim-sulphamethoxazole (Septrin), NSAIDS, penicillins
High risk patients	Old age, renal impairment, alcohol (>7 units per week), body weight >40% above normal, diabetes mellitus

NSAIDs, non-steroidal anti-inflammatory drugs.

presence of normal liver function tests.[202] Hypersensitivity pneumonitis occurs in up to 10% of patients on methotrexate for rheumatoid arthritis.[193]

Contra-indications (Table 3.8). Both pregnancy and conception should be avoided within six months of treatment of either partner, because methotrexate is teratogenic.[194] Breast feeding is also contra-indicated. Co-administration of other antifolate agents such as trimethoprim-sulphamethoxazole (Septrin) may increase the toxic effects of methotrexate on the bone marrow, as may non-steroidal anti-inflammatory drugs, penicillin, old age and renal impairment. To reduce the risk of hepatotoxicity, methotrexate should not be prescribed to patients who drink more than seven units of alcohol/week, weigh over 40% greater than normal or have diabetes mellitus.[201]

Monitoring treatment. The risks of bone marrow depression necessitate weekly full blood counts for four weeks then every one to two months, with folic acid co-administration at a dose of 1–5 mg/day.[200] Liver function tests including albumin should be monitored every one to two months. Liver biopsy is probably unnecessary except in patients with persistently abnormal liver function tests or after a cumulative dose of more than 5 g.[202] Unexplained shortness of breath or cough necessitates a chest radiograph and blood gases and lung function tests, particularly carbon monoxide diffusing capacity.[193] It is possible to measure methotrexate blood levels; however, in practice these provide little benefit, as levels predict neither efficacy nor toxicity.[198]

Limitations. Although North American trials indicate that methotrexate may have a useful role in patients with steroid-refractory or steroid-dependent Crohn's disease,[195,199] there remain unanswered questions. The minimum effective dose is not yet clear. Oral administration of methotrexate appears to increase gastrointestinal side-effects, particularly soon after dosing, but would be preferable to injections if proved efficacious. Indeed, a trial of enteral versus parenteral administration would be helpful.

It is not clear exactly when methotrexate should be used, although most gastroenterologists resort first to a thiopurine rather than methotrexate in steroid-resistant or steroid-dependent patients. Evidence is also required about the relative merits of methotrexate and thiopurines when given in combination with infliximab (see below).

Mycophenolate mofetil

Mechanism of action. Mycophenolate mofetil is an ester prodrug, widely used to prevent rejection of renal transplants. It appears to act by reducing lymphocyte proliferation by inhibiting inosine monophosphate dehydrogenase and thus synthesis of guanosine nucleotides,[203] and cytokine release.[204]

Indications. Several preliminary studies,[205–207] and an unblinded, single-centre comparative trial[204] have suggested that mycophenolate might prove a useful alternative to azathioprine, acting more quickly and being at least as well tolerated. However, two uncontrolled studies have failed to confirm this proposal.[208,209]

Side-effects. Side-effects include nausea, weight gain, headache and insomnia. Opportunistic infections such as cytomegalovirus, herpes simplex and candidiasis have been reported as has drug-related colitis.[210] Bone marrow depression and hepatitis necessitate blood monitoring similar to that recommended for thiopurines and methotrexate. Mycophenolate may carry a higher risk of lymphoma when given long term than azathioprine.[206] Pregnancy should be avoided until at least six weeks after the end of treatment.

Limitations. In the absence of a definitive controlled trial to assess the efficacy and safety of mycophenolate it is difficult at present to justify the use of this relatively expensive drug in the management of Crohn's disease.

Ciclosporin A

Mechanism of action. Inhibition of IL-2 gene transcription by ciclosporin reduces helper- and cytotoxic T-cell function.

Preparations. In acute severe ulcerative colitis, the intravenous preparation is given at 4 mg/kg per day as a continuous infusion to ensure rapid achievement of therapeutic blood levels.[211] The levels are checked at 24 hours and held at 250–400 ng/ml to maximize therapeutic effect and minimize side-effects. After the patient has been stabilized with the intravenous preparation, treatment is usually continued as oral ciclosporin. The original oral preparation, Sandimmun (5–8 mg/kg per day), is variably and frequently poorly absorbed, especially in the presence of intestinal inflammation. Neoral, the newer oral preparation, is better absorbed. Trough levels should be in the range 150–300 ng/ml.

Indications. Although it has become a valuable adjunctive therapy in steroid-refractory acute severe ulcerative colitis,[211] a role for ciclosporin in achieving or maintaining remission in Crohn's disease is not yet established. An early controlled trial showed some benefit from using a high dose of oral ciclosporin (5–7.5 mg/kg per day) for three months for active disease.[212] However, remission was not maintained in these patients (who did not receive continuing ciclosporin).[213] Further studies have failed to show benefit from ciclosporin at lower doses (5 mg/kg per day); in particular, any possible therapeutic improvements were counterbalanced by side-effects.[214,215] As a result, ciclosporin is not recommended as routine treatment for Crohn's. The only possible current indications for ciclosporin may be refractory perianal fistulae (Chapter 6) and acute severe Crohn's colitis in pregnancy as an attempt to avoid surgery.[216]

Side-effects. The many serious side-effects of ciclosporin are summarized in Table 3.9.[217]

Table 3.9 Side-effects of and contra-indications to ciclosporin.[312]

Side-effects

General	Nausea, vomiting, headache
Renal	Interstitial nephritis
Infection	Opportunistic including *Pneumocystis carinii* pneumonia
Neurological	Epileptic fits, parasthesiae, myopathy
Hypertension	
Skin	Hypertrichosis, gingival hypertrophy
Metabolic	Hyperkalaemia, hypomagnesaemia, hyperuricaemia
Liver	Cholestatic hepatitis
Malignancy	Lymphoma

Contra-indications

Pregnancy and lactation	
Disease	Renal impairment, hypertension, infection, epilepsy, malignancy
Biochemical	Low serum cholesterol or magnesium, high potassium
Drugs	Co-administration of cytochrome P450 inhibitors (grapefruit, erythromycin, oral contraceptives, fluconazole, calcium channel and proton pump inhibitors) Co-administration of cytochrome P450 inducers (phenytoin, barbiturates, rifampicin, carbemazepine, St John's wort)

(Reproduced from Rampton. In: Rampton (ed.) *Inflammatory Bowel Disease, Clinical Diagnosis and Management.* London: Martin Dunitz Ltd, 2000[312] with permission from Martin Dunitz.)

Contra-indications. The risk of fits contra-indicates the use of ciclosporin in patients with low serum magnesium and/or cholesterol concentrations. Co-administration of cytochrome P450 inhibitors such as grapefruit juice, the oral contraceptive pill and proton pump inhibitors may lead to toxic blood levels of ciclosporin (Table 3.9). Cytochrome P450 inducers (phenytoin, rifampicin and carbamazepine) may decrease ciclosporin levels, as may St John's wort, an alternative therapy widely used for treatment of depression.[218] Other contra-indications to ciclosporin are shown in Table 3.9.

Monitoring treatment. Strict alternate day monitoring of serum levels of ciclosporin is required during intravenous therapy, together with daily monitoring of renal function and serum magnesium and potassium levels. When the patient is switched to oral medication, the trough level of ciclosporin, renal and liver function, serum magnesium and potassium, urate and cholesterol levels should be checked weekly for a month then at least monthly.[217]

Limitations. There is as yet no clear indication for the use of ciclosporin in Crohn's disease, and its adverse safety profile makes it unlikely to become a major therapeutic player in this setting.

Tacrolimus (FK506)

Tacrolimus is a macrolide, with similar mode of action and side-effects to ciclosporin. Unlike ciclosporin, it is well absorbed orally even from inflamed gut; it is also more potent. Preliminary reports suggest that it may be useful for patients with difficult perianal or fistulating disease, either alone or in conjunction with a thiopurine or corticosteroid.[219-221] The oral dose is about 0.1–0.3 mg/kg per day to give a serum concentration of 10–20 ng/ml.[219] Topically applied tacrolimus paste may heal oral ulceration due to Crohn's.[222] Neurotoxicity and nephrotoxicity are more common after oral tacrolimus than ciclosporin; cardiomyopathy and impaired glucose tolerance can also occur. Minor side-effects include diarrhoea, flushing, nausea, headache and tremor.[219]

The toxicity of tacrolimus makes it an unlikely candidate for widespread application in patients with Crohn's disease, even if proven to be efficacious.[220]

Cyclophosphamide

Preliminary data suggest that intravenous cyclophosphamide (750 mg, four to six cycles at monthly intervals) may be effective in refractory Crohn's disease, but controlled data are required to assess its possible role.[223]

Anti-TNF therapies

Anti-TNF-α antibody (infliximab)

Mechanism of action. Infliximab acts by binding to free TNF-α (a pro-inflammatory cytokine) (Chapter 1) as well as TNF-α bound to the surface of activated T-cells. Membrane-bound infliximab mediates complement activation and subsequent antibody-dependent cytolysis of the inflammatory cells; it also leads to their caspase-dependent apoptosis by increasing the ratio of BAX to Bcl-2.[224] The cytokine cascade is consequently down-regulated and recruitment of lymphocytes into the intestinal mucosa is reduced.[225,226]

Preparations. The only preparation currently available for routine clinical use is infliximab (Remicade), a cA2 mouse–human chimeric antibody. It is given as an intravenous infusion over two hours, either once only or at intervals (see below) at a dose usually of 5 mg/kg.[227] Depending on the weight of the patient, the cost of each such infusion is about £1500 (US $2200).

A 95% humanized antibody, CDP571, has been developed but will not become routinely available.[228,229] This antibody is less immunogenic than infliximab; it also binds to membrane-bound TNF-α but fails to induce complement-dependent cytolysis.

Indications. In refractory active Crohn's disease, a single infusion of 5 mg/kg infliximab produced an improvement in about 60% of patients, compared with 20% given placebo; remission occurred in 33% of patients treated compared with 4% of those on placebo.[227] Benefits lasted 8–12 weeks and clinical improvement on infliximab was associated with healing of mucosal appearances and disappearance of the mucosal inflammatory infiltrate.[120] A later trial showed that repeated infusions of infliximab maintained remission over the course of a year in 62% of patients, compared with 37% of those given placebo.[230] These findings have been extended in a much larger study (ACCENT I) in which it was also found that infliximab reduced steroid usage.[231]

Safety and cost considerations (see below) suggest that the use of infliximab should be restricted to patients with severe Crohn's, which is refractory to treatment with corticosteroids, aminosalicylates, antibiotics, liquid formula diet and immunomodulatory drugs, or where there has been intolerance to or toxicity from these treatments.[232] Additionally, patients to be given infliximab should have usually been deemed inappropriate for surgery, for example because of the risk of inducing short bowel syndrome (Chapter 9).

The only controlled trials of infliximab in fistulous Crohn's disease to date have related primarily to perianal rather than enterocutaneous and other fistulae.[115,233] In the first trial, successful healing, indicated by a reduction of drainage from most perianal fistulae, was reported in 60% of patients given three infusions of infliximab in six weeks, compared with 26% of those given placebo.[115] However, the median duration of response was only three months and about 10% of infliximab-treated patients developed abscesses. MRI scanning showed that infliximab tended to heal the openings of fistulae rather than the tracts themselves.[234] In the ensuing ACCENT II trial,[233] further infliximab at 5 mg/kg given at eight-week intervals for a year maintained complete healing in 36% of patients (vs 19% for placebo). Non-responders to this dose of infliximab often improved when given 10 mg/kg; 15% of patients developed abscesses related to their fistulae and rectovaginal fistulae responded particularly poorly.

Taken together these trials mitigate against the use of infliximab for fistulous Crohn's disease except in patients with concurrent chronically symptomatic disease elsewhere in the GI tract.[232,233,235]

Strong evidence-based recommendations cannot yet be made about the advisability of concurrent therapy with thiopurines or methotrexate. However, as in rheumatoid arthritis, it is likely that coprescription of such drugs will improve efficacy, and/or reduce the dosage and/or toxicity of infliximab.[236–238] Indeed, early experience indicates that coadministration of a thiopurine increases the time to relapse and reduces infusion reactions in patients given infliximab for Crohn's, effects likely to be a consequence of reduced production of antibodies to infliximab (ATI).[191] Conversely, it is conceivable that coprescription of infliximab with other immunosuppressants could increase the risk of opportunistic infections and lymphoma.[239]

Although clinical experience is even more limited than in adults, children may benefit from treatment with anti-TNF antibody, particularly if this permits a reduction in corticosteroid use and an increase in bone mass and growth (Chapter 8).

Controlled data relating to anti-TNF therapy other than infliximab are limited. The humanized monoclonal antibody, CDP571, is efficacious in patients with otherwise refractory Crohn's.[228,229,240] On the other hand, a recent trial indicates that etanercept, a recombinant TNF-receptor fusion protein, is ineffective in Crohn's disease, a result contrasting with that obtained in rheumatoid arthritis[241] and possibly explained by the failure of etanercept, unlike infliximab, to bind to membrane-bound TNF and thereby induce T-cell apoptosis.

Side-effects. Common side-effects associated with the infusion itself include headache, rash, nausea and fever (Table 3.10). These are usually mild and respond to antihistamines, but anaphylaxis may occur and antihistamines, adrenaline and corticosteroids should be available when infusions are given.

Several infections have been described in patients given infliximab, of which the most serious is tuberculosis.[242,243] Infliximab-related reactivation of tuberculosis occurs in about 1/2000 patients,[242] is commonly miliary and has caused more than 100 deaths worldwide to date; it is an unsurprising adverse effect in view of the importance of TNF-α in controlling intracellular infections.

Infliximab can exacerbate congestive cardiac failure.[244] Neurological complications of infliximab have also been reported: they include aseptic meningitis[245] and irreversible de novo demyelination as well as exacerbation of multiple sclerosis.[246]

In patients with pre-existing intestinal strictures, particularly if fibro-stenotic rather than inflammatory, rapid healing by fibrosis may precipitate bowel obstruction.[247]

There are isolated reports of lymphoma in patients given infliximab for Crohn's disease or rheumatoid arthritis, but it is not yet clear whether these are due to the drug itself or to concurrent therapy with immunosuppressive agents or whether they are a complication of the underlying disease.[239]

Although contra-indicated in pregnancy (see below), the outcome of unintended pregnancies in patients given this treatment for rheumatoid arthritis and Crohn's disease has been satisfactory.[248]

Repeating infusions of infliximab after an interval longer than 20 weeks[249] increases the risk of development of antibodies to infliximab (ATI, formerly known as human antichimeric antibodies (HACA)). These may reduce the efficacy of infliximab,[191,250] and can cause a serum sickness-like reaction characterized by myalgia, arthralgia, rash and fever which responds to

Table 3.10 Side-effects of and contra-indications to infliximab.

Side-effects

General	Headache (20%), nausea (10%), upper respiratory tract infection (10%)
Serious infections	Tuberculosis, salmonella, cellulitis, pneumonia (including *Pneumocystis carinii*), histoplasmosis, listeriosis, aspergillosis, coccidioidomycosis, candida
Infusion reactions	Headache, rash, nausea, fever
Intestinal	Obstruction
Autoantibodies	Antibodies to infliximab (ATI), anti-DNA and cardiolipin antibodies with lupus syndrome
Malignancy	Lymphoma (possibly)
Congestive cardiac failure	
Neurological	Aseptic meningitis, demyelination, exacerbation of multiple sclerosis

Contra-indications

Pregnancy and childbirth either current or planned in the next six months
Breast feeding
Failure to use contraception
Active infections, sepsis
Intestinal strictures
Previous tuberculosis
Congestive cardiac failure
Multiple sclerosis
Current or previous malignancy
Hypersensitivity to mouse proteins
Prolonged interval between infusions   Risk of ATI and serum sickness

(Reproduced from Rampton. In: Rampton (ed.) *Inflammatory Bowel Disease, Clinical Diagnosis and Management*. London: Martin Dunitz Ltd, 2000[312] with permission from Martin Dunitz.)

prednisolone and analgesics, but may contra-indicate further infliximab.[251] Early data suggest that intravenous hydrocortisone given prior to infliximab,[252] and thiopurines given long term,[191] may reduce formation of ATI.

Antibodies to double-stranded DNA and to cardiolipin have been seen in up to 15% of patients given infliximab for Crohn's disease and a transient lupus syndrome has been reported in those with rheumatoid arthritis.[253]

Contra-indications. Exclusion criteria are shown in Table 3.10. Previous tuberculosis requires exclusion with a detailed history and a chest radiograph. Unfortunately, the high incidence of anergy restricts the usefulness of tuberculin skin testing in patients with Crohn's.[254,255] In patients needing infliximab who have a history of TB and/or a chest radiograph indicating previous infection, co-administration of isoniazid is recommended.[242,256]

The pharmacokinetics of infliximab in the elderly and in patients with renal or liver disease is insufficiently clear to allow recommendations about treatment. Lastly, the manufacturers suggest that to minimize the risk of ATI (HACA), infliximab should not be given as retreatment after an interval of 15 weeks, although recent data suggest that 20 weeks might be a more pragmatic cut off.[249]

Monitoring treatment. Prior to therapy, potential contra-indications (Table 3.10) require meticulous exclusion (see above). During the infusion and for one hour afterwards, patients should have half-hourly pulse, blood pressure, respiratory rate and temperature measurements. The risk of anaphylaxis means that infusions should be given in hospitals with full resuscitation facilities available. Patients on courses of infliximab need careful clinical follow-up, looking particularly for evidence of side-effects such as tuberculosis.

Conclusions. Infliximab was the first specifically targeted biological therapy to reach the bedside for the treatment of Crohn's disease: how it should be used has been well-reviewed recently.[251]

Early experience suggests that non-smokers, young patients, those with Crohn's colitis and those already on immunosuppressive therapy are most likely to respond to anti-TNF antibody. However, more data are needed to identify patients less likely to benefit: clearly these should not be exposed to the potential side-effects and costs of treatment if possible. At present, it is suggested that patients failing to respond to a maximum of two infusions should not be offered further infliximab, but in future, non-responsive individuals may be predictable by their genotype.[108,109,257]

Further trials are required to define optimal treatment regimens, but to evaluate dose, frequency, duration and concurrent therapy in the various different clinical presentations of Crohn's disease will be an enormous task.

Thalidomide

Thalidomide reduces the production of TNF-α and IL-12,[258] and has been evaluated in small, open clinical trials for refractory Crohn's disease. It appears to be modestly effective in doses of 50–300 mg/day, decreasing the need for corticosteroids, healing mucosal lesions and fistulae.[259] A particular role may be in treating oral and difficult upper gastrointestinal Crohn's disease.[259,260] Its potential application, however, will be restricted by its side-effects. Thalidomide is of course teratogenic, causing phocomelia and other abnormalities. Patients need to practise abstinence or use two forms of contraception with regular testing for pregnancy before and during treatment.[259] Other serious side-effects include drowsiness, peripheral neuropathy, oedema and dermatitis.[259]

Other anti-TNF approaches

Onercept is a recombinant human TNF-receptor p55 monomer thought to act by neutralizing soluble TNF: it was efficacious in a preliminary open-label trial in active Crohn's.[261] CDP870, a pegylated humanized FAB fragment to TNF[697] and adalimumab, a fully humanized Ig4 antibody to TNF are also under evaluation.[698] CNI-1493 is a small molecule that blocks TNF gene expression by inhibiting the MAP kinase signalling pathway. A preliminary study suggests that, given intravenously, it is worth further trial in active Crohn's.[262]

Future developments in therapy

Recent advances in our understanding of the immune response, inflammatory process and cellular biology (Chapter 1) have led to the assessment in animal models, and in many instances in human patients, of a wide range of new agents designed to act at specific pathophysiological targets (Figure 3.5); in reality their mode of action is often likely to be more complex than indicated by the classification shown in Table 3.11. Approaches that have reached clinical trial in patients with Crohn's disease are described below.

Modifying gut luminal flora

Increasing evidence points to a pivotal role for normal gut flora in driving the mucosal immune and inflammatory response in patients with IBD (Chapter 1). Modification of the microbial flora for therapeutic gain has been attempted by feeding patients with bacteria thought to have a protective or

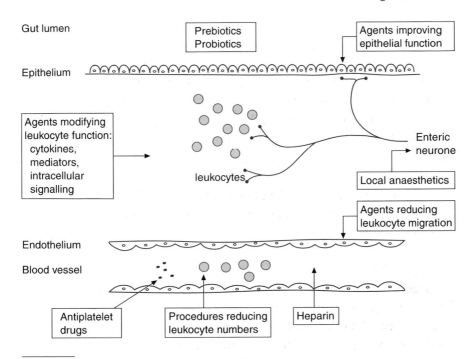

Gut lumen

Prebiotics
Probiotics

Agents improving
epithelial function

Epithelium

Agents modifying
leukocyte function:
cytokines,
mediators,
intracellular
signalling

Enteric
neurone

leukocytes

Local anaesthetics

Agents reducing
leukocyte migration

Endothelium

Blood vessel

Antiplatelet
drugs

Procedures reducing
leukocyte numbers

Heparin

Figure 3.5 *Schematic representation of possible sites of action of novel therapies for Crohn's disease.*

anti-inflammatory role, 'probiotics',[17,33] and with parasites designed to alter the immune response in a favourable direction.[263] Possible mechanisms of action of probiotics include production of antimicrobial factors, competitive interactions with pathogens and modification of epithelial permeability and signalling and of the mucosal immune response.[33] Lastly, genetically engineered probiotic bacteria can be used to deliver anti-inflammatory compounds to inflamed mucosa, an approach already tried in mice using IL-10-secreting *Lactococcus lactis*.[264]

The beneficial effects of enteral feeding (Chapters 5 and 9) may be achieved at least in part through changes in gut bacterial flora, but studies of the potential therapeutic benefits in Crohn's disease of 'prebiotic' food constituents, such as inulin,[265] given to induce specific changes in intestinal flora, have not yet been reported.

Probiotic therapy

Treatment with capsules containing non-pathogenic *E. coli* may reduce relapse rate in UC,[266,267] while a gastric acid-resistant cocktail (VSL#3) of eight

Table 3.11 Potential new treatments for Crohn's disease.[312]

Target	Agent
Colonic bacterial flora	Probiotics
	Saccharomyces boulardii
	Trichuris suis eggs
Epithelium	Growth hormone
Leukocytes	
• Reduce numbers	Apheresis
	Anti-CD4 antibodies
	Bone marrow transplant
	Stem cell transplant
• Reduce migration	ICAM-1 antisense
	Alpha 4-integrin antibody
• Modify function:	
Stimulate granulocytes	GCSF, G-MCSF
↓ Pro-inflammatory cytokines	Onercept, RDP58, anti-IL-12 antibody
↑ Anti-inflammatory cytokines	IL-10, IL-11
↓ Soluble mediators	Ridogrel, SOD, GTN, fish oil
Modify intracellular signalling	NFκβ antisense, PPARγ agonist, MAPK inhibitor
Agents targeting enteric neurones	Local anaesthetics
Modulation of procoagulant state	Heparin

ICAM, intercellular adhesion molecule; GCSF, granulocyte colony stimulating factor; G-MCSF, granulocyte-macrophage colony stimulating factor; IL, interleukin; SOD, superoxide dismutase; GTN, glyceryl trinitrate; NFκβ, nuclear transcription factor κβ; PPARγ, peroxisome proliferators activated receptor-γ; MAPK, mitogen-activated protein kinase.

organisms, including various strains of bifidobacteria and lactobacillus, appears efficacious in pouchitis.[268] In a small study, *Saccharomyces boulardii* improved the efficacy of 5-ASA in preventing relapse of Crohn's.[269] The results of ongoing controlled European trials of the effects of probiotics in Crohn's disease are keenly awaited. Long-term toxicity studies will be needed to ensure that probiotics do not have unsuspected side-effects, such as systemic sepsis in the event of mucosal translocation, transference of antibiotic resistance and colorectal carcinogenesis. In this context, there has been a report of liver abscess after use of a probiotic lactobacillus species.[270]

Improving gut epithelial function

Short-chain fatty acids

Although benefit has been claimed for the use of enemas containing short chain fatty acids in UC,[271,272] there are no studies of the use of topical short-chain fatty acids in Crohn's disease.

Growth hormone

In a preliminary report, the CDAI of patients given subcutaneous growth hormone injections with a high protein diet improved more than those given placebo and the same diet.[273] How growth hormone may work in Crohn's is unclear, but its effects include increased mucosal uptake of amino acids and electrolytes, reduced gut permeability and increased gut protein synthesis. These results need confirmation; fears of the tumorigenic potential of growth hormone must also be allayed.

Reducing leukocyte numbers

Uncontrolled reports have shown that reduction of circulating leukocyte numbers by leukocyte apheresis,[274] allogeneic bone marrow transplant[275] or autologous stem cell transplantation[276] suppresses activity of Crohn's disease. Depletion of CD4-positive T-cells using a chimeric monoclonal anti-CD4 antibody also appears to reduce CDAI in patients with otherwise refractory Crohn's,[104,277] an effect mirroring that which has been reported in patients with both Crohn's and HIV as the CD4 count falls.[278,279] Any of these procedures, however, would seem to be potentially too toxic, as well as expensive, for use except in exceptionally refractory Crohn's disease.

Reducing leukocyte migration

Two agents designed to reduce egress of leukocytes from blood vessels into the intestinal mucosa have undergone clinical trial in Crohn's.

ICAM-1 antisense oligonucleotide

ICAM-1 (intercellular adhesion molecule-1) plays a central role in leukocyte adherence to and migration through capillary endothelia. Pilot data suggesting that an antisense oligonucleotide to ICAM-1 (ISIS 2302) was efficacious in patients with active Crohn's were not confirmed in two larger placebo-controlled studies.[280,281]

Alpha 4-integrin antibody

Like ICAM-1, alpha 4-integrins are important mediators of the migration of leukocytes, particularly lymphocytes and monocytes, across vascular endothelia. In a pilot trial, a single infusion of natalizumab, a recombinant humanized monoclonal antibody to alpha 4-integrin, reduced CDAI in patients with moderately active Crohn's.[282] In a subsequent larger study, two infusions of natalizumab were more effective than placebo in inducing improvement (73% vs 38%), remission (46% vs 27%), reduction in C-reactive protein and a decrease in endoscopic disease activity.[283] As anticipated, these changes were associated with increases in circulating T and B lymphocytes; side-effects were rare. Natalizumab clearly needs further investigation in Crohn's disease.

Modifying leukocyte function

Methods used experimentally to modify leukocyte function in patients with Crohn's disease include:

- Stimulating granulocytes
- Antibodies to pro-inflammatory cytokines
- Anti-inflammatory cytokines
- Agents inhibiting the synthesis or antagonizing the receptors of soluble inflammatory mediators
- Agents which modify intracellular signalling.

Stimulating granulocytes

Intestinal damage resembling that of Crohn's disease occurs in chronic granulomatous disease and glycogen storage disease; improvement follows therapy with granulocyte colony stimulating factor (GCSF) and granulocyte-macrophage colony stimulating factor (G-MCSF). Preliminary work suggests a potentially beneficial role for these compounds in Crohn's[284] and a phase II trial using G-MCSF is in progress.

Down-regulating the effects of pro-inflammatory cytokines

The use of infliximab has been described above. Undergoing clinical trial in both Crohn's and UC is an orally administered small protein, RDP58, which has been shown to reduce TNF-α production and inflammation in an animal model of IBD.[285] Trials are in progress to assess the effects of antibodies to other pro-inflammatory cytokines, including IL-12.[286]

Anti-inflammatory cytokines

The mucosal immune response is modulated by anti- as well as by pro-inflammatory cytokines.[46]

Interleukin-10. IL-10 is a regulatory cytokine which inhibits both antigen presentation and release of pro-inflammatory cytokines[287] and seemed to have substantial therapeutic potential in inflammatory gut disease.

Several placebo-controlled clinical trials have shown that intravenous or subcutaneous injections of IL-10 (Tenovil) produced only a very modest clinical response in active Crohn's.[288–290] It was also ineffective in preventing postoperative recurrence of Crohn's in a placebo-controlled trial.[291] In the short term, the only overt side-effects of IL-10 have been a reversible anaemia and thrombocytopenia, but if IL-10 were to achieve long-term systemic usage there would be a concern about the risks of infection and neoplasia.

At present the development of this regulatory cytokine for parenteral treatment of IBD has been suspended.[104] However, there remains interest in stimulating its release in the gut mucosa by topical application of an adenoviral gene vector[287] or in orally administering an IL-10-secreting genetically engineered lactococcus.[264]

Interleukin-11. Recombinant human IL-11, like IL-10, antagonizes Th1 cytokines. Two placebo-controlled trials suggest that this cytokine is effective in active Crohn's, inducing remission in 37% vs 16% of patients on placebo,[292,293] but a further trial was stopped after an unfavourable interim analysis.[104]

Antagonizing inflammatory mediators

Lipid mediators. Reducing synthesis of pro-inflammatory prostaglandins with non-selective NSAIDs has an adverse rather than beneficial effect in IBD, perhaps because of the concomitant suppression of cytoprotective prostaglandins.[34] Selective COX-2 inhibitors appear to have a deleterious effect in animal models of IBD[294] and seem unlikely to undergo evaluation as treatment for Crohn's disease.

Trials with inhibitors of the synthesis of the potent leukocyte chemo-attractant leukotriene B4 were disappointing in UC,[295] but have not been undertaken in Crohn's disease. Ridogrel inhibits the synthesis and antagonizes receptors of thromboxane A2, but a placebo-controlled trial failed to show any benefit in moderately active Crohn's disease.[296]

Reactive oxygen species. While increased mucosal production of reactive oxygen species in IBD is well established,[49] published trials of antioxidant therapy in Crohn's are limited to one open study of patients with steroid-refractory disease who appeared to benefit from intramuscular superoxide dismutase.[297] A small trial showed no benefit from oral enteric-release glyceryl trinitrate,[298] given as a nitric oxide donor.

Fish oil. Eicosapentaenoic acid (EPA), the active ingredient of fish oil capsules, decreases synthesis of eicosanoids, platelet activating factor and IL-1. One trial in Crohn's was entirely negative.[299] However, an enteric-coated fish oil preparation, which is better tolerated than standard formulations, has been reported to reduce the relapse rate in patients with inactive Crohn's.[300] This interesting result needs confirmation.

Modulating intracellular signalling

New insights into the mechanisms controlling intracellular signalling have raised the possibility of developing further agents to inhibit mucosal inflammation in IBD.[48]

The first of these to reach clinical trial is an antisense oligonucleotide to the p65 subunit of NFκβ, a nuclear transcription factor playing a central role in the pathogenesis of inflammation. To date this approach has been applied only in a limited trial of topical therapy of distal IBD.[15,301,302]

Other potentially beneficial agents acting on intracellular signalling targets include a peroxisome proliferators activated receptor-γ (PPARγ) agonist[303] and mitogen-activated protein (MAP) kinase inhibitor.[262]

Agents targeting enteric neurones

Abnormalities of the enteric nervous system have been identified in patients with IBD (see Figure 1.2).[6] Topical local anaesthetics appear to be effective in uncontrolled studies in proctitis,[304] but have not been assessed in Crohn's disease.

Modulation of procoagulant state

Patients with Crohn's show evidence of a procoagulant state, with abnormalities of clotting factors, thrombocytosis and increased platelet activation

(Chapter 9).[53] As indicated above however, treatment with ridogrel, which inhibits platelet aggregation, had no benefit in Crohn's.[296]

Heparin
Heparin has a range of anti-inflammatory as well as anticoagulant actions.[305,306] Several small studies have suggested that intravenous heparin might be of therapeutic value in UC,[305] although at least one controlled study has given negative results.[307]

There is very limited information on the use of heparin in Crohn's colitis[308,309] and properly designed controlled trials would be needed before the use of heparin could be justified in this disease.

Supportive drugs

Antidiarrhoeals
Diarrhoea in patients with Crohn's disease has several mechanisms (see Table 2.2), each requiring diagnosis and specific treatment.

Symptomatic treatment with antidiarrhoeal drugs may additionally be necessary. The most frequently used preparations are codeine phosphate (30–240 mg/day), loperamide (2–16 mg/day) and Lomotil (1–6 tablets/day). These drugs should be avoided in active Crohn's colitis in case they induce toxic dilatation.[310] Other side-effects include constipation, abdominal pain and bloating. Codeine phosphate may induce dependency.

Bile salt binding agents
In patients with extensive ileal disease or resection, bile salt malabsorption may cause watery diarrhoea. Although bile salt malabsorption can be confirmed using a SeHCAT isotope scan,[90] it is usually reasonable to give bile salt binding agents such as cholestyramine or colestipol sachets (4 g bd up to 12 g bd) empirically. However, in patients with extensive ileal disease or resection (greater than 100 cm), treatment-induced bile salt depletion may worsen steatorrhoea.[311] Furthermore, cholestyramine and colestipol may reduce absorption of other nutrients (for example, vitamin K and folic acid). They may also bind other medications and should be given more than two hours before or after any other therapy. Some patients find these agents unpalatable.

chapter 4

Principles of surgical management of Crohn's disease

Introduction

Surgery in Crohn's overcomes only its complications; it is not curative. Most patients with Crohn's require surgery eventually, up to 90% having to undergo surgery by 30 years after onset of symptoms.[55,314] Furthermore, the high rate of postoperative recurrence of Crohn's leads to the need for repeated surgical intervention at a rate of about 5% per year.[315] Hence, surgery for patients with Crohn's disease should be undertaken as part of a strategic plan for their management.

Indications for surgery

The common indications for surgery are shown in Table 4.1.[67] Patients with small bowel Crohn's disease usually require surgery for obstruction or

Table 4.1 Indications for surgery in Crohn's disease.

Recurrent intestinal obstruction
Intestinal perforation ± fistula and abscess formation
Gastrointestinal bleeding; acute or chronic
Perianal disease
Intractable disease
Growth failure (children)
Toxic megacolon
Small or large bowel cancer
Extraintestinal manifestations

perforation, while those with colonic Crohn's are usually operated on for failure to respond adequately to medical therapy.

In paediatric practice patients with growth failure often show 'catch-up' growth after surgical resection (Chapter 8).[316]

Principles of surgical intervention

The guiding principles of surgical intervention are:

- Elective surgery should not be performed without an adequate trial of medical management.
- The goal of surgical intervention is palliation of symptoms and restoration of health.
- Surgical intervention should be safe: it should carry minimal morbidity and no mortality.
- Surgical intervention should preserve as much of the gastrointestinal tract as possible. Repeated surgery due to recurrent disease is common: repeated resection of wide margins of normal bowel can cause short bowel syndrome (Chapter 9).
- Surgical intervention should be undertaken as soon as there are appropriate indications.

Preoperative considerations

Baseline documentation of the extent of the patient's disease, including small bowel barium studies and colonoscopy (Chapter 2), should be obtained. CT scanning in patients with suspected sepsis allows accurate definition of any abscess, allows preliminary percutaneous drainage and may prevent the later requirement of a stoma.

Metabolic deficiencies require assessment and correction. Patients who are malnourished may benefit from preoperative parenteral nutrition (Chapter 5).[317] However, it may be difficult to restore nutritional deficiencies in patients with a protein-losing enteropathy and response may occur only after resection of the diseased bowel. It is important to identify those patients with low-grade intra-abdominal sepsis in whom a delay of surgery for attempted nutritional correction may be detrimental, especially as the benefit of preoperative nutrition is unproven.[318] For patients currently on or who recently received steroid therapy, hydrocortisone (100 mg) intravenously every six to eight hours is given to cover perioperative stress.

Bowel preparation may be given to patients without intestinal obstruction undergoing large bowel resection electively. All patients who may require a stoma should be counselled preoperatively by a stoma therapist.

Surgical treatment of Crohn's disease at specific sites

The sites most commonly requiring surgery for the complications of Crohn's disease are the ileum, colon and rectum, and anorectum.

Small bowel disease

Up to 40% of patients undergoing surgery have small bowel and ileocaecal Crohn's.[319] They commonly present with obstructive symptoms or with sepsis secondary to perforation and intra-abdominal abscess formation with or without intestinal fistulae (Table 4.1).

Surgical resection

Ileocaecal disease is usually managed by resection, particularly when surgery is being performed for the first time. The diseased bowel is thick and fibrotic, with fat wrapping, mesenteric thickening and adenopathy (Figure 4.1).

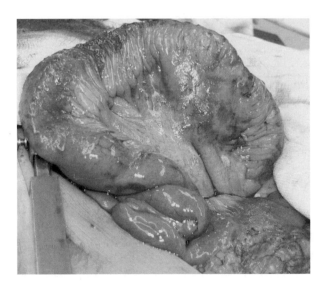

Figure 4.1 *Crohn's disease of the terminal ileum showing the classical appearance of fibrotic bowel wall, fat wrapping, mesenteric thickening and adenopathy.*

Although Crohn's almost always involves the terminal ileum, proximal skip lesions are found in up to 20% of cases. Mucosal and submucosal lesions may not be seen without careful inspection. Subtle strictures can be identified by passing a Foley catheter into the lumen of the bowel through an enterotomy, threading the bowel on to the catheter, inflating the balloon of the catheter and drawing the catheter back along the bowel. The diameter of the stricture can be assessed by measuring the maximum diameter of the balloon that can be pulled through it.

Ileal Crohn's disease should be excised with grossly disease-free margins at the proximal and distal ends. Whilst early reports recommended wide disease-free margins,[320] more recent studies have shown that narrower margins of excision do not lead to an increase in recurrence rates.[321] At the Cleveland Clinic, 131 patients prospectively randomized to resection with narrow or wide (2 cm or 12 cm) margins showed no significant difference in clinical recurrence rate or the need for further surgery.[321] Recurrence rates were also similar irrespective of whether the resection margins were histologically healthy or microscopically involved with Crohn's disease.[321] Current surgical practice is for limited resection with 2–3 cm macroscopically disease-free margins on either side of the diseased segment.

Skip lesions close to major areas of involvement in the terminal ileum can be resected in continuity. However, when the length of bowel involved in skip lesions or continuous lesions is great, the surgeon is faced with an operative dilemma. Total excision of all gross disease may risk causing short bowel syndrome. Partial excision, however, would leave active, symptomatic disease behind. The possible strategies for dealing surgically with extensive small bowel disease are discussed in the next section.

In patients with a single stricture, a primary anastomosis is usually constructed, with or without a covering stoma, after surgical resection. The orientation of the anastomosis and whether it is fashioned with sutures or staples do not appear to affect the risk of recurrence.[322,323]

In general, anastomosis should be avoided in the presence of major intra-abdominal sepsis. However, an anastomosis can be performed in an otherwise healthy patient with localized sepsis providing the site of anastomosis lies well away from the septic focus.

There are no absolute indications for constructing a protective stoma following resection for small bowel Crohn's. Healing may be compromised in patients who are malnourished, on long-term steroid or immunosuppressive therapy or have intra-abdominal sepsis. These patients, as well as those who have had difficult surgery with multiple small bowel interventions, may require diversion proximal to an anastomosis. It is often best to fashion a loop ileostomy or jejunostomy proximal to the site of disease with a view to definitive surgical resection three to six months later when the patient is in a better nutritional state.

Recurrences usually occur at or just proximal to the anastomosis, but reported recurrence rates following resection for small bowel Crohn's disease vary widely. This is at least in part because recurrences can be defined in clinical, radiological, endoscopic, histological or surgical terms (Chapters 2 and 3).

Asymptomatic recurrence can be identified endoscopically soon after resection. Rutgeerts et al found endoscopic recurrence in 72% of patients within a year of operation.[324] The earliest sign of recurrence was aphthous ulceration near the resection margins. Although these sites do not predict the sites of later symptomatic disease, symptoms are more likely to develop in patients with severe recurrent disease found on imaging.[325]

Symptomatic recurrence occurs in about 6% of patients per year, or in 30% at 5 years and 60% at 10 years.[67] Recurrence rates are greater when multiple sites of Crohn's disease are present.[326] Other risk factors for recurrent disease are outlined in Chapters 2 and 3.

Repeat resections for small bowel Crohn's disease are needed in 15–45% of patients by five years after primary surgery.[67,327] Following a second operation for Crohn's disease, the rates of recurrence are similar to those following the initial one.

Management of extensive small bowel disease

There are two options available for dealing surgically with multiple skip lesions or long contiguous segments affected by Crohn's disease.

Exclusion bypass. In the early years of surgery for Crohn's, a complicated adherent mass in the ileocaecal region was often treated by a bypass procedure. The involved segment was bypassed with a side-to-side anastomosis between uninvolved proximal small bowel and adjacent colon. Although this operation preserved small intestine and bypassed symptomatic lesions, it left diseased and often partially obstructed bowel in situ. Because of this and the risk of later neoplastic change in the excluded segment of bowel (Chapter 9), bypass procedures are rarely performed today.

Strictureplasty. Strictureplasty was first described in 1982[328] and it effect-ively widens the lumen at the sites of narrowing without removing any intestine. The procedure involves making longitudinal incisions through the narrowed segments of bowel and closing the incisions in a transverse direc-tion, the Heineke–Mikulitz strictureplasty (Figure 4.2). The Finney type stric-tureplasty (Figure 4.3) may be used for multiple or confluent strictures.

(a)

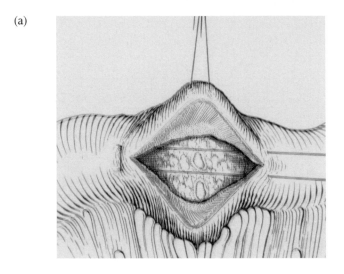

(b)

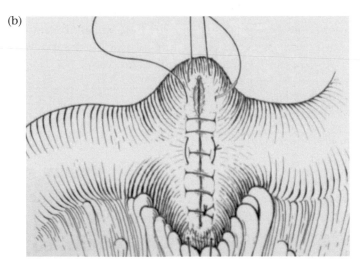

Figure 4.2 *Short strictureplasty (Heineke–Mikulitz). (a) A longitudinal enterotomy is made over the strictured segments of the small bowel. (b) This is then closed transversely to widen the stenotic segment of bowel.*

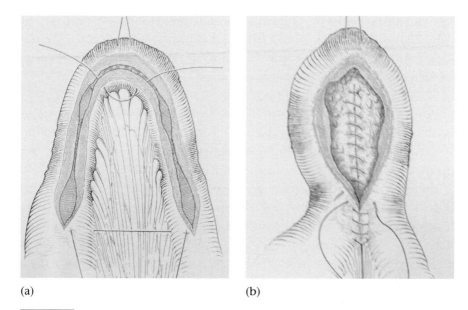

(a)   (b)

Figure 4.3 *Long strictureplasty (Finney). Multiple adjacent or confluent strictures are all opened longitudinally from normal bowel proximally to normal bowel distally (a). The incised bowel is then bent over in a loop and the posterior wall is sutured with a continuous seromuscular suture. The seromuscular suture is then continued along the anterior wall of the loop of bowel (b).*

Strictureplasty is most useful in patients with multiple short strictures over long segments of intestine and in those who have already had several previous resections and are at risk of short bowel syndrome (Chapter 9). Strictureplasty can also be used for short uncomplicated primary strictures, ileocolic or ileorectal anastomotic strictures, recurrent stricturing at sites of previous strictureplasties and duodenal strictures.

Strictureplasty is contra-indicated in patients with active sepsis or fistula or in malnourished patients in whom closure of the enterotomy carries a risk of anastomotic dehiscence. The presence of a solitary stricture close to other segments for which resection is planned is also a relative contra-indication.

Experience with strictureplasty has been excellent. Recent data from Oxford over a 15-year period on 52 patients who had 241 strictureplasties showed no mortality.[329] Postoperative sepsis occurred in only 4% of cases. Thirty-six per cent of patients required a second operation after 1–57 months. The majority of recurrences were in new segments of obstructing or perforating disease. Site-specific recurrence occurred at nine (4%) strictureplasty sites in four patients. The cumulative reoperation rates after first and second strictureplasty were identical, with a four-year reoperation rate of 30%. The reoperation rate when strictureplasty was used alone or in combination with resection was found to be similar, being 35–40% at five years. These results are similar to those of the largest series from North America.[330]

Endoscopic balloon dilatation. For the minority of patients in whom small bowel strictures are accessible to an enteroscope or colonoscope, endoscopic balloon dilatation using a hydrostatic balloon is a relatively non-invasive therapeutic option (see also Chapter 6, Figure 6.3).

There are as yet no controlled data to assess the efficacy and safety of this approach. However, in the largest published case series of endoscopic balloon dilatation in 55 patients with Crohn's disease, 59 ileocolonic strictures were dilated a total of 78 times.[331] Complete and long-term relief of obstructive symptoms was reported in 60% of patients, of whom a third needed two or more dilatations to achieve this result. Ten per cent of patients incurred perforations, although only two of these needed surgical rather than conservative management. The value of concurrent local mucosal injection of corticosteroids such as triamcinolone is not yet proven.[332,333]

Surgical management of small bowel fistulae in Crohn's disease
Fistulae caused by Crohn's often involve other intestinal segments and organs, usually with an associated abscess. They occur in about 35% of patients with Crohn's.[334] The most common types of fistulae are entero-enteric and enterocolonic (Table 4.2). Although isolated enteroenteric fistulae are usually asymptomatic unless associated with obstruction or sepsis, when managed non-surgically 40% of patients require surgery within a year and a further 33% within 10 years.[327] Hence most patients, unless at high risk of complications resulting from repeated surgery, should be advised to undergo definitive surgery for their fistulous disease.

Surgery for fistulae is dependent on the anatomic site involved (Table 4.3). The aim of the operation is to eradicate the obstructing disease associated with the fistula. In general, the source is resected, the target structure repaired and the bowel anastomosed to restore intestinal continuity. Faecal diversion is used selectively after bowel anastomosis.

Table 4.2 Intestinal fistulae in Crohn's disease.[334]

	No of fistulae (%)
Enterocutaneous	46 (16)
Enteroenteric (including enteroduodenal)	65 (23)
Enterocolonic	83 (29)
Enterosigmoid	49 (17)
Enterovcsical	36 (12)
Enterovaginal	4 (4)
Enterosalpingeal	2 (2)
Colosigmoid	5 (2)

Total number of patients = 639.
Number with fistulae at 290 sites = 222.

Table 4.3 Management of common enteric fistulae in Crohn's disease.

Source of fistula	Target organ	Management of fistula source	Management of target organ
Ileum	Ileum or jejunum	Resection	Primary closure or resection if unable to close
Ileum	Skin	Resection	Debridement
Ileum	Colon	Resection	Primary closure or resection if unable to close
Ileum	Duodenum	Resection	Primary closure or duodenojejunostomy if unable to close
Ileum	Bladder	Resection	Debridement and primary closure
Ileum	Vagina	Resection	Debridement and primary closure
Colon	Ileum or jejunum	Resection (colectomy)	Primary closure or resection if unable to close

Management of intra-abdominal sepsis

Free bowel perforation. In this unusual situation, patients present with generalized peritonitis and circulatory failure. The most common pathology is free perforation proximal to partially obstructed terminal ileum with release of small bowel contents into the peritoneal cavity. Management consists of aggressive fluid and electrolyte resuscitation prior to laparotomy.

At surgery, peritoneal toilet is performed and the obstructed and perforated segment of bowel is resected. In patients with ileal perforation who present early, a primary anastomosis may be used selectively. If the colon has perforated, primary anastomosis is inadvisable. The same is true in those patients with small bowel perforation who have longstanding peritonitis, are immunocompromised, are malnourished or have failure of one or more organ: a proximal ileostomy with distal mucous fistula is advisable in such situations.

Localized intra-abdominal abscess. The majority of abscesses arise from ileal Crohn's disease. They may be complicated by an inflammatory phlegmon, sometimes with a fistula to another loop of bowel. Retroperitoneal perforation may cause a psoas abscess, on the right in patients with ileal disease and on the left in the less common patients in whom the descending or sigmoid colon is the source of the abscess. The clinical manifestations vary from mild sepsis to severe psoas spasm with hip pain, flexion deformity and external rotation of the thigh associated with an abdominal mass.

The recommended management is image-guided drainage, antibiotic therapy and elective resection of the diseased segment once sepsis has resolved. This approach often avoids the need for a stoma. Primary surgical intervention may be required in situations where image-guided drainage is ineffective or inappropriate, such as the presence of multiloculated abscesses. In this situation, laparotomy with drainage of the abscess and resection of the diseased bowel is preferred. A primary anastomosis may be performed if it is distant from the site of sepsis.

Duodenal disease

Duodenal Crohn's disease is uncommon (Chapter 2) and almost always associated with ileal disease. It usually results in duodenal obstruction, but perforation with fistulae into the pancreas and peripancreatic tissue may also occur. Treatment is primarily medical (Chapter 6); strictures can be dilated endoscopically (Chapter 6).[335]

When surgery is required, gastrojejunostomy rather than duodenal resection is preferred, although duodenal strictureplasty has been performed in selected patients. Controversy exists on the use of vagotomy to prevent marginal ulceration. The incidence of the latter is low (<5%) and some investigators feel that it does not justify the morbidity of postvagotomy diarrhoea. Furthermore, marginal ulceration can often be managed satisfactorily with medical therapy.[336]

Colonic and rectal Crohn's disease

About two-thirds of patients with large bowel Crohn's disease require surgical intervention. The operation rate is highest for those patients with right-sided involvement, largely because these patients tend to have co-existing ileal disease that requires ileocolic resection. The lowest operation rate is in patients with rectal disease only.

The surgical management of Crohn's disease of the large bowel varies, depending on the sites of involvement and the severity of the disease (Table 4.4).

Segmental colectomy

Patients with localized segments of large bowel inflammation and a normal rectum can sometimes be managed by segmental resection and primary end-to-end anastomosis. The advantage of this procedure is the avoidance of a stoma. Continence and frequency of defaecation are generally satisfactory. However, recurrence rates of up to 62% at five years[337] and reoperation rates of 66% at 10 years have been reported.[338]

Table 4.4 Surgical options for large bowel Crohn's disease.

Sphincter preservation with restoration of intestinal continuity	Segmental colectomy Total colectomy and ileorectal anastomosis ?Ileal pouch–anal anastomosis – controversial
Sphincter preservation with diverting stoma	Diverting ileostomy Total colectomy and ileostomy
Resection of bowel and anal sphincters	Total proctocolectomy and ileostomy

Total colectomy and ileorectal anastomosis

Patients with severe disease of the colon but mild or minimal rectal disease (25–50% of patients with large bowel Crohn's disease) should have a total colectomy and ileorectal anastomosis.[339] In healthy patients, a one-stage procedure is performed. Patients with significant comorbidity may undergo two-stage surgery with an initial diverting ileostomy and closure of the rectal stump followed by later restoration of intestinal continuity.

The advantage of ileorectal anastomosis is that the source of chronic protein-losing colitis or sepsis is eradicated and a stoma or perineal wound is avoided. For young women particularly, the social, sexual and marital advantages of this are considerable. However, at least 50% of these patients eventually require rectal excision.[339]

Ileorectal anastomosis should not be performed in emergencies because a primary anastomosis in this setting is associated with a high anastomotic leak rate. A good functional result and a low risk of early rectal excision are largely determined by patient selection: the procedure is not advisable, for example, in the presence of rectal inflammation, active perianal disease, a rigid, non-distensible rectum, rectal dysplasia or cancer.[340]

A satisfactory result is achieved in 65% of patients undergoing ileorectal anastomosis.[339] Cumulative recurrence rates vary from 38% at five years to 74% at 10 years.[341,342] Not all recurrences require operation, reoperation rates in patients with recurrent disease varying from 25 to 66%.[341,342] Although the recurrence rate is partly related to concomitant ileal disease, perianal disease has a major impact on the need for subsequent rectal excision.

Ileal pouch–anal anastomosis

Unlike ulcerative colitis, ileoanal pouch construction is not generally recommended for patients with Crohn's since it usually results in recurrence of inflammation in the pouch, fistulae at the anastomosis and peripouch abscesses. However, despite efforts to diagnose patients preoperatively correctly with either Crohn's disease or UC, some patients undergo pouch surgery only to have a subsequent histological diagnosis of Crohn's disease made on the colectomy specimen. Although controversial, the results of such inadvertent pouch formation in patients with Crohn's colitis in published series are not as unfavourable as commonly believed. Good functional results in 65% of such cases over a three-year period have been reported,[343] whilst one group of investigators has reported a pouch failure rate of only 45% over a 10-year period despite disease recurrence in 92% of pouches.[344]

Diverting ileostomy

Diverting ileostomy, leaving the large bowel in place, is seldom used now. The procedure may have a role in patients who are severely ill with Crohn's colitis and unable to tolerate extensive surgery. The goal of ileostomy is to minimize morbidity, facilitate colonic and perianal healing, allow for a more limited future resection and possibly delay proctocolectomy.[345] However, continued disease activity requiring treatment usually follows this procedure. Patients with diverting ileostomies may eventually have their stomas closed, but colonic disease often flares up after closure. Most eventually undergo proctocolectomy and permanent ileostomy.

Total colectomy and ileostomy

This procedure involves removal of the colon, formation of an end ileostomy and closure of the proximal rectum, leaving the rectum and anal canal in place but excluded from the faecal stream. It is the best procedure in patients who are poor candidates for proctocolectomy, including those with toxic colitis, toxic megacolon, or significant comorbidity. It is also recommended in patients with severe colonic disease and mild rectal disease, but with anorectal problems such as fistulae or abscess. Preservation of the rectum also allows patients with indeterminate colitis to avoid inappropriate ileoanal pouch surgery while reserving this option if a diagnosis of UC is later established. Persistent or recurrent anorectal disease, seen in 70% of cases, is the most common indication for later excision of the rectum and anus.[346] Haemorrhage, perforation and cancer are further indications. Rectal excision may also be indicated when endoscopic or radiological surveillance of the bowel is difficult, as with a rectal or anal stricture.

Total proctocolectomy and ileostomy

Total excision of the colon, rectum and anus with formation of a permanent end ileostomy is the best procedure for patients with severe involvement of the colon and rectum. Defective perineal wound healing occurs in about a third of patients.[315] Recurrence of Crohn's disease in the small bowel after this procedure ranges from 3 to 46%:[347] recurrent disease usually involves the distal ileum within 25 cm of the ileostomy.[348]

Surgical management of anorectal disease

Although seldom the only sites of disease, the anus and rectum are involved in 8–90% patients with Crohn's disease (Chapter 2).[349,350] The prevalence range is wide because of variability in classification and the thoroughness with which the search for such lesions is conducted. Over 50% of patients with colonic involvement have anal complications, as compared to less than 20% of patients with small bowel disease.[351]

The common anorectal manifestations in Crohn's disease are listed in Table 4.5. A thorough clinical examination including rectal examination will diagnose most anorectal abnormalities. However, some patients will require examination under anaesthesia for painful conditions and when perianal sepsis is present. For more complex presentations, additional investigations such as barium studies, fistulography, CT scanning with rectal contrast, endorectal ultrasound and MRI may be required (Chapter 2).

Surgical management of anorectal Crohn's disease should be as conservative as possible. Wide excisions should be avoided. With conservative medical and surgical therapy, symptoms are often improved; abscesses, fistulae and fissures may heal, particularly in the absence of colonic disease.

Abscesses – ischiorectal and perianal

The prevalence of abscesses in patients with anorectal Crohn's disease is about 50%.[352] These abscesses may be complex and multiple and often have to be evaluated radiologically. Surgical drainage is the treatment of choice. Recurrent abscesses occur in only about one-half of patients during the two

Table 4.5 Anorectal manifestations of Crohn's disease.

Abscesses – Perianal and ischiorectal
Fissures
Anal skin tags
Haemorrhoids
Fistula-in-ano
Proctitis
Ulcers
Strictures
Incontinence
Rectovaginal fistula
Cancer

years following the initial drainage,[353] so additional examination for a potential fistula-in-ano is rarely performed acutely. However, in patients with recurrent abscesses, the likelihood of concurrent fistulae is high and a rigorous search necessary.

Anal fissure

Anal fissures in Crohn's disease are usually deep, indolent, relatively painless and in the midline. The fissures are usually self-limiting.[354] Even if symptomatic, most fissures can be treated medically with topical agents such as 0.2% glyceryl trinitrate ointment, with only 15% requiring surgical intervention.[355] Painful fissures are usually associated with underlying sepsis and require examination under anaesthesia. If an abscess is found, drainage with internal lateral sphincterotomy provides symptomatic relief without leading to incontinence.

Anal skin tags and haemorrhoids

Anal skin tags are usually asymptomatic and only present problems when they interfere with perianal hygiene. About 25% resolve spontaneously, particularly after remission of underlying bowel disease.[352] Asymptomatic skin tags should not be excised unless malignancy is suspected, as this may result in an unhealed wound, anal ulcer or perianal sepsis.

Management of symptomatic haemorrhoids should be conservative. Dietary manipulation and the use of topical medications are usually successful. If patients remain symptomatic, injection or rubber band ligation of the haemorrhoids should be considered. Surgery is reserved for the few patients with severe symptoms, such as those with persistent prolapsed and bleeding haemorrhoids and those with thrombosed haemorrhoids. Postoperative complications include perianal sepsis, anal stenosis, fistula and unhealed wounds. Some of these may eventually lead to rectal and anal excision.

Fistula-in-ano

Management of anorectal fistula-in-ano may be challenging in Crohn's disease. The danger is poor healing and the development of faecal incontinence after overly aggressive surgery. Fistulotomy (deroofing and laying open of the fistula) and drainage of any associated perianal sepsis should be the first-line treatment of simple low-lying fistulae. Healing rates of 60–75% have been reported.[356,357] Fistulae that do not heal often have co-existing perianal sepsis, are complex or have rectal involvement. If involvement of the anal sphincter is suspected, two alternatives to fistulotomy are insertion of a seton and performance of a rectal mucosal advancement flap.

A seton is a non-absorbable suture or vessel loop made of silicone rubber. This is passed through the cutaneous opening of the fistula, into the lumen of the anal canal and then back out to the skin surface, where it is tied loosely to itself. The intervening skin and mucosa are trimmed away under the seton. The seton maintains a patent external opening to the fistulous tract and thereby controls local sepsis. It may be left in place for varying amounts of time, even as much as a year, and should not be removed until disease is quiescent.

Patients with proctitis and low-lying fistulae may have problems after fistulotomy, with healing rates of only about 50%.[358] Medical therapy is usually helpful (Chapters 3 and 6). High-lying or complex fistulae present the most difficult scenario and are best managed with setons and medical therapy. However, up to 20% of patients may still require excision of the rectum and anus.[359]

Stricture

Anorectal strictures may be due to inflammation, abscesses, fistulae and ulcers.[360] About 50% occur in the rectum, 33% in the anus and the remainder in the anorectum. They may result in a diaphragmatic deformity or be long and tubular. Most occur in patients with co-existent proctitis or perianal disease.

Most strictures are asymptomatic or self-limiting, but some cause incontinence, urgency, tenesmus and difficulty in evacuation. Medical treatment with topical 5-ASA preparations, steroids and antibiotics may be useful. Short, particularly diaphragmatic strictures may be amenable to digital or endoscopic balloon dilatation (see above and Chapter 6). However, many symptomatic strictures require faecal diversion or excision of the rectum and anus.

Faecal incontinence

Faecal incontinence is a common and distressing problem in patients with anorectal Crohn's disease, occurring in up to 40% of cases.[361] The cause is multifactorial and may be secondary to severe, chronic fibrosis and scarring of the anorectum with loss of reservoir function. In this situation either faecal diversion or excision of the rectum and anus is indicated. Similarly, faecal diversion is indicated in severe Crohn's-related anal sphincter destruction; it may also be necessary in patients with profuse diarrhoea and incontinence from colitis or short bowel syndrome.

Laparoscopic surgery in Crohn's disease

Surgery for inflammatory bowel disease in general, and Crohn's disease in particular, can be challenging even for the most experienced surgeon using conventional techniques. Laparoscopic management may be attempted according to the level of skill and experience of the surgeon. The threshold for conversion to an open procedure should be low. Patient selection is of the utmost importance and early experience should be confined to uncomplicated cases. Thin, rather than obese patients and patients with segmental as opposed to diffuse disease should be selected.

The role of laparoscopic surgery in Crohn's disease is still being evaluated. There are very few data available (Table 4.6), most of which are from small series of laparoscopic ileocolic resections in selected patients with primary uncomplicated disease. In general, the results are good, with a mean morbidity of 5%, a hospital stay of five days and conversion rates of 11%. One of the largest series has demonstrated that, contrary to popular opinion, laparoscopic-assisted surgery can be accomplished safely in the presence of localized abscess, phlegmon or recurrent disease around a previous anastomosis.[362]

Table 4.6 Laparoscopic surgery for Crohn's disease.

No of patients	Procedure	Conversion rate (%)	Theatre time (min)	Morbidity	Mean hospital stay (days)	Reference
9	IC resection	0	170	0	7	366
20	Mixed	0	NS	0	NS	367
25	IC resection	24	NS	NS	6	363
18	IC resection	0	105	6	5	368
31	Mixed	29	195	4	6	364
49	Mixed	14	144	14	5	365
46	IC resection	11	144	7	4	362

IC, Ileocolic; NS, not stated.

Other reported procedures undertaken laparoscopically include small bowel resection, strictureplasty, subtotal colectomy, segmental colectomy, panproctocolectomy and gastrojejunal bypass.[363–365] Results of subtotal colectomy and proctocolectomy have been less good than those of ileocaecal resection, with increased morbidity and longer operating times and hospitalization. Furthermore, laparoscopic total colectomy does not appear to offer any advantages over the conventional open approach.[365]

The feasibility and safety of laparoscopic surgery in the management of selected patients in Crohn's disease have been proven. However, only prospective randomized studies of laparoscopic versus conventional open surgery in patients with similar disease extent and indications for surgical intervention can truly compare both modalities.

chapter 5

Nutritional and other approaches to the treatment of Crohn's disease

Introduction

This chapter discusses the place of nutritional therapy and the importance of abstaining from smoking; it concludes with a section on the use of complementary therapy by patients with Crohn's.

Nutrition as primary therapy

Enteral nutrition plays a small but important role in the treatment of Crohn's in adults, being particularly useful in those suffering troublesome side-effects from drugs. It is most useful in children, in whom both active disease and corticosteroids cause growth failure (Chapter 8).

Mechanism of action

The original aim of using nutrition as a primary therapy was to allow 'bowel rest', either using an enteral diet absorbed proximally in the small bowel, leaving minimal residue to pass into disease-affected areas, or bypassing the gut completely using total parenteral nutrition (TPN). Proposed mechanisms of action of nutritional therapy now also include reductions in epithelial permeability, mucosal secretion and exposure to food antigens, together with changes in gut flora and mucosal immunity.[369] These mechanisms may also depend indirectly on the positive effect of nutritional repletion on nitrogen balance.

Total parenteral nutrition (TPN)

Several, but not all retrospective uncontrolled trials have suggested a benefit from TPN as sole treatment for active Crohn's.[370-374] Furthermore, prospective studies have shown no difference between the effects of TPN alone and polymeric diet or partial TPN combined with enteral feeding.[375,376] Current evidence therefore indicates no advantage in using TPN as primary therapy for active Crohn's. Furthermore, the expense and complications of TPN therapy far outweigh those of enteral feeding.

These comments do not exclude the use of TPN as a supportive therapy, for example in the perioperative period (Chapters 4 and 6) or in patients with short bowel syndrome (Chapter 9).

Enteral nutrition

Preparations

The many liquid enteral feeds available differ in their composition, antigenicity, palatability and site of absorption in the intestine. All these diets are complete, containing constituents of proteins, carbohydrates and fat, as well as essential trace elements and vitamins (Table 5.1).

Monomeric feeds are unpalatable but less antigenic than other diets, and their high content of glutamine may theoretically be trophic to gut mucosa.[369] However, in practice, the use of glutamine-enriched feeds confers no advantage, at least in children.[377] Elemental diets reduce gastrointestinal protein loss[378] and improve gut permeability in Crohn's.[379] Diets containing larger molecular weight polypeptides require a greater length of bowel for absorption and may be more antigenic; whether this is of practical importance has not been proven (see below).

Indications

Controlled trials of enteral feeding to date have compared different diets with each other or with corticosteroids, but none has been placebo-controlled. Many have been insufficiently blinded. The results in some trials have been inappropriately interpreted on a per protocol, rather than intention-to-treat basis, an important consideration because of the high drop-out rate of patients given enteral therapy. The number of patients in several trials is small. Other problems in trial interpretation include selection bias, variable length of treatment and a high recurrence rate in the months after discontinuation of enteral feeding.[380]

Table 5.1 Constituents of enteral diets.

Diet	Example	Example constituents
Monomeric or elemental diet	Elemental 028 – powder or in cartons (3 g amino acids, 11 g carbohydrate, 3.5 g fat with 1550 kJ/100 ml)	Amino acids, sugars (short-chain maltodextrins and glucose) and fatty acids
Oligomeric diets	Perative – nasogastric feed (6.7 g protein, 17.7 g carbohydrate, 3.7 g fat with 551 kJ/100 ml)	Protein constituents as peptides or protein hydrolysates
Polymeric feeds	Fresubin – sip feed or via nasogastric tube (3.8 g protein, 13.8 g carbohydrate, 3.4 g fat with 420 kJ/100 ml)	Whole proteins

Adapted from reference 369.

Meta-analyses have concluded that enteral nutrition produces clinical remission in about 60% of patients, compared with about 70% of those given corticosteroids, and that there is no clear difference in the efficacy of different preparations.[25,26] Trials to test the proposal that diets low in long-chain triglycerides (LCT) may be more effective than those providing a high percentage of energy as LCT,[381] have given conflicting results.[382,383] Furthermore, the proposal that a liquid diet containing growth factor (Modulin-IBD) might be particularly effective[384] has yet to be confirmed in a controlled trial. An open study does, however, suggest that a transforming growth factor β_2-containing feed induces mucosal healing and down-regulates mucosal pro-inflammatory cytokines in children with Crohn's (Chapter 8).[385]

By comparison with corticosteroid and other pharmacological therapy, enteral nutrition, at least in adults, has a limited role in view of its poor palatability, tolerability and expense. In well-motivated individuals, however, it can prove a very useful and safe therapy where drug side-effects have been troublesome. Additionally, enteral therapy continues to have an important adjunctive role in improving nutrition in sick patients with extensive Crohn's disease.

Side-effects

Many patients do not tolerate enteral feeds because of their taste. Some will not persist with nasogastric feeding if this is necessary to maintain feed volumes. Other side-effects include diarrhoea, which can usually be averted by gradually increasing the daily intake of feed, electrolyte imbalance, reactive hypoglycaemia and infection.

Monitoring

A full nutritional assessment prior to starting enteral nutrition is required so that, where necessary, specific deficiencies can be rectified. Initially, twice weekly nutritional variables (see Table 9.4) as well as laboratory markers of disease activity should be measured; frequency is decreased as therapy continues.

Conclusions

The relative merits of enteral feeds of differing composition require further analysis in controlled trials. It is still not clear exactly how such therapy works, nor whether efficacy varies with site of disease. Lastly, it remains unclear how best to reintroduce conventional food after enteral feeding. The Cambridge group serially introduce a selected range of foods, excluding in the long term those which produce symptoms.[27] However, the efficacy of exclusion diets has not yet been confirmed elsewhere and most gastroenterology services, in the UK at least, have insufficient dietetic support for this type of dietary management.

Stopping smoking

The evidence for smoking as a causative agent in Crohn's disease is outlined in Chapter 1. A recent prospective, interventional study found that for patients who stopped smoking, the risk of relapse over a two-year period was significantly lower than in those who continued smoking and resembled that of non-smokers.[24] The need for corticosteroids and immunosuppressives was increased in continuing smokers.[24] Factors increasing the likelihood of smoking cessation were the particular physician responsible for the patient, previous intestinal surgery, high socio-economic status and the use of oral contraceptives.[24] In other studies, smokers with Crohn's have been found to have the same willingness to quit as the rest of the population.[386]

Complementary and alternative therapy

The terms complementary and alternative medicine denote theories and practices in medicine which deviate from the conventional, the former when they are applied as an adjunct to and the latter when they are used instead of standard management. The combined term comprises a heterogeneous range of diagnostic and therapeutic procedures ranging from traditional practices such as acupuncture, traditional Chinese medicine, homeopathy and herbal medicine, to more modern complementary practices including aromatherapy and reflexology.

Current usage

Recent surveys have shown that up to 50% of people in the Western world use complementary therapy.[387] Similarly, approximately half of patients with gastrointestinal disorders including IBD have used complementary therapy, most commonly herbal remedies.[388-391] The widespread usage of complementary therapy in IBD is likely to be related to its chronic and refractory nature[389] and has been linked with poor quality of life in relation to psychosocial function.[391]

Efficacy

Limited data suggest that Boswellia serrata and some traditional Chinese medicines may have efficacy in UC,[218] but there are none on the efficacy of complementary therapies in Crohn's. Despite the difficulties associated with evaluating complementary medicine,[392] it is essential, in view of the widespread usage of complementary approaches by patients with Crohn's, that efforts are made to assess scientifically the efficacy and safety of, at least, those therapies most frequently used.

Side-effects

While it is unlikely that therapies such as reflexology will have direct adverse effects, the same cannot be said of herbal therapies, toxicity from which has included fatal liver as well as irreversible renal failure.[218]

The interaction of herbal therapies with conventional drugs needs further clarification. In the context of Crohn's, however, St John's wort reduces blood levels of ciclosporin by enhancing the activity of cytochrome P450 enzymes, while gingko, ginger and devil's claw reduce absorption of orally administered iron.[218]

Perhaps more importantly, use of complementary therapies may be complicated by indirect adverse effects. For example, patients initially consulting alternative practitioners may suffer from misdiagnosis. Others may delay or forego appropriate conventional options in favour of ineffective unconventional ones.

Conclusions

There is an urgent need for further scientific assessment of the benefits and dangers of complementary therapy, in IBD, as for other applications. Herbal preparations, in particular, should require licensing by an independent national body in order to improve their quality and safety and to ensure that claims of efficacy are validated by controlled trials. The general public, pharmacists and doctors need to be aware of the direct and indirect risks associated with the use of complementary therapies.

chapter 6

Management of specific clinical presentations of Crohn's disease

Introduction

The approaches to the treatment of the different intestinal problems arising in patients with Crohn's disease are described in this chapter. Treatment of Crohn's disease depends on its site, activity and the pathological process underlying the patient's symptomatology.

Determination of disease activity and of need for hospital admission

Its heterogeneous presentation prevents the assessment of disease activity in Crohn's disease from being straightforward. Multi-factorial clinical and/or laboratory-based scoring systems, such as the CDAI[97] and Harvey–Bradshaw index[98] (Chapter 2), are unsuitable for ordinary clinical use,[76,122] and the working definitions of the American College of Gastroenterology are more practicable (Table 6.1).[122]

Most patients with active Crohn's can be looked after as outpatients, but those with severe disease need prompt hospital admission. In patients with Crohn's colitis, indications for admission resemble those for acute severe UC, for example six or more diarrhoeal stools daily, pyrexia, tachycardia, anaemia and/or weight loss.

Table 6.1 Working definition of disease activity in Crohn's disease.[122,312]

Activity	Features
Remission	Asymptomatic patients
Mild-moderate	Outpatients able to take oral nutrition, with symptoms but no fluid depletion, fever, abdominal tenderness, painful mass or obstruction
Moderate-severe	Patients who have failed to respond to treatment of mild-moderate disease or those with more prominent symptoms including fever, weight loss >10%, abdominal pain or tenderness (without rebound), intermittent nausea or vomiting (without obstructive findings) or anaemia
Severe-fulminant	Patients with persisting symptoms despite outpatient oral steroids or those with a high fever, persistent vomiting, intestinal obstruction, rebound tenderness, cachexia or abscess

Management of active Crohn's disease

General principles

The key aspects of the management of active Crohn's are summarized in Table 6.2.[312]

Diagnosis

To establish the site of disease and the pathological processes causing the first presentation or relapse, a range of investigations is required (Chapter 2) (Table 6.3). Not every patient will require all investigations, particularly when the site of disease has previously been established. However, it is essential to clarify the presenting pathology to optimize subsequent treatment.

Team organization

A multi-disciplinary team approach involving, at least, a medical and surgical gastroenterologist, a gastrointestinal radiologist and histopathologist, dietitian and specialist IBD nurse is essential for optimal management of Crohn's. Decisions about management should be made in close conjunction with the patient so that he/she can play an informed part in therapeutic decisions.

Table 6.2 General management of active Crohn's disease.[312]

General measures	Explanation, psychosocial support Patient support groups (NACC) Specialist multi-disciplinary care with physicians, surgeons, nutrition team, IBD nurse, stoma therapists, counsellor
Establish diagnosis, severity, and extent/site	Clinical evaluation Investigations as in Table 6.3
Monitoring progress	Daily clinical assessment Stool chart Four-hourly temperature, pulse Alternate day FBC, ESR, C-reactive protein, urea and electrolytes, albumin Daily plain abdominal radiograph (if patients acutely unwell or with obstruction or severe colitis) Weekly weight
Supportive treatment	Fluids, electrolytes, blood transfusion Nutritional supplements, low residue diet in presence of small bowel stricture Haematinics (B_{12}, folate, iron) Analgesia, antidiarrhoeals (not in acute situation) Prophylactic heparin Avoid NSAIDS, delayed-release drugs

Specific treatment (separately or in combination)	*Medical*
	  Corticosteroids (intravenous or oral)
	  High dose 5-ASA if already taking, otherwise start in recovery phase
	  Consider metronidazole, clarithromycin, ciprofloxacin; broad-spectrum antibiotics if sick or febrile, or evidence of infection/abscess
	  Azathioprine/6-mercaptopurine/methotrexate if steroid-unresponsive
	  Anti-TNF antibodies (infliximab) for non-responders to steroids and immunomodulators
	Nutritional
	  Liquid formula diet
	Endoscopic
	  Balloon dilatation of strictures
	Surgical
	  Resection or strictureplasty

Table 6.3 Investigations to identify the site and define the pathology of relapses of Crohn's disease.

Type of investigation	Specific tests	Indications
Blood tests	FBC, ESR, C-reactive protein, urea and electrolytes, ferritin, B_{12}, folate, LFT, Ca^{2+}, Mg^{2+}	Evidence of acute phase response/sepsis/ malnutrition or malabsorption
Stool microbiology	Culture, microscopy, *Clostridium difficile* toxin	To exclude enteric infection
Endoscopy, biopsy	Colonoscopy/flexible sigmoidoscopy, including biopsies for TB culture	Right iliac fossa pain or mass, diarrhoea, rectal bleeding
	OGD and duodenal biopsies	Upper gastrointestinal symptoms
Radiology	Plain abdominal radiograph	Symptoms of obstruction or mass in right iliac fossa; to estimate disease extent or severity in Crohn's colitis
	Barium studies	To establish disease site and fistulous connections
	Radiolabelled leukocyte scan	To identify sites of bowel inflammation and intra-abdominal sepsis
	Ultrasound, CT or MRI scanning	To establish sites of disease and allow percutaneous drainage of abscesses

FBC, full blood count; ESR, erythrocyte sedimentation rate; LFT, liver function tests; OGD, oesophagogastroduodenoscopy; MRI, magnetic resonance imaging; CT, computerized tomography; Ca^{2+}, calcium; Mg^{2+}, magnesium; TB, tuberculosis.

Explanation, education and psychosocial support

Newly diagnosed patients need a full explanation of their disease. Written information should be given with local hospital contact numbers in case of relapse. Leaflets from patient support groups such as the National Association for Colitis and Crohn's disease (NACC) are written with patients and their carers in mind (see Appendix). They include information about not only medical and surgical treatment options, but also cancer risk, pregnancy, controversial issues such MMR (measles, mumps, rubella) vaccination and practical problems ranging from travel overseas through life insurance to filling in social security forms. The NACC also runs local support groups which can benefit patients by putting them in touch with others in their neighbourhood.

Being given a diagnosis of Crohn's disease may have major psychological consequences[393,394] and some patients require formal psychosocial help (Chapter 9).

The availability of a specialist IBD nurse (Chapter 10) allows many queries to be answered less hurriedly and without the pressures patients often feel when attending a busy medical outpatient clinic. If surgery is planned, and particularly when a stoma is possible, prior access to a stoma care nurse is essential to allow full discussion of its implications.

Dietary advice

Patients should be advised to take a balanced diet containing adequate nutrients including, for example, calcium to help prevent osteoporosis (Chapter 9).

Patients with known small bowel stricturing should be given a low residue diet sheet to reduce the chances of episodes of obstruction. Such diets avoid high residue foods such as sweetcorn, celery, nuts and pulses.

In patients with steatorrhoea, a low fat diet often reduces bowel symptoms. Occasionally replacement of long-chain by medium-chain triglycerides is necessary (Chapter 9).[369] The value of specific exclusion diets for the treatment of Crohn's disease is unconfirmed.[27] However some patients do claim that individual foods provoke symptoms, and it is reasonable that they exclude these items from their diets.

Nutritional support in patients with chronic or severe diarrhoea

Water and electrolyte balance require careful monitoring, with replacement of fluids and electrolytes intravenously or orally as appropriate.

Nutritional status should be checked with appropriate haematological and biochemical blood tests (see Chapters 5, 9 and 10, Table 9.4), together with measurement of height and weight. This allows calculation of the body mass index (BMI) (weight in kilogrammes divided by (height in metres)^2). Active nutritional intervention is needed if the BMI falls below 20 or if the weight falls by more than 10% within a two-month period (Chapter 9).

Supportive drug therapy

Chronic diarrhoea needs evaluation as indicated in Chapter 2. Many patients with chronic diarrhoea will need loperamide or codeine phosphate; those with bile salt malabsorption will usually benefit from cholestyramine and those with small bowel bacterial overgrowth from antibiotics (Chapter 3).

Because of the risk of thromboembolic disease (Chapter 9), subcutaneous heparin is recommended for patients admitted with active Crohn's.[395] Treatment of other complications of Crohn's disease, such as anaemia and osteoporosis, is described in Chapter 9.

Drugs to avoid

NSAIDs predispose to relapse of IBD and should be avoided if possible.[34] Anti-diarrhoeal agents should be avoided in patients with acute severe Crohn's colitis because of the risk of provoking acute colonic dilatation.[396] Delayed release drugs may precipitate intestinal obstruction in patients with stricturing small bowel disease.

Specific treatment

The principles of the specific treatment of active Crohn's disease are outlined in Table 6.4 and Figure 6.1. Treatment can be pharmacological, nutritional, surgical and/or endoscopic. Every patient should be advised to stop smoking.[24]

Patients with mildly active disease can be started on a 5-ASA, for example Pentasa,[139] or an antibiotic such as ciprofloxacin[159] or metronidazole.[152] Patients with moderately active inflammatory disease (Table 6.1) are usually given an oral corticosteroid. If the presentation is with severe or fulminant disease, admission to hospital is required (Table 6.1): intravenous steroids are often necessary in patients without major sepsis (see below).

Patients responding well to steroids are generally weaned off them in two to four months. There are no proven therapies for the maintenance of medically-induced remission of Crohn's disease other than abstinence from smoking.

In patients who fail to respond to steroids, or who relapse when the dose of steroids is reduced or soon after discontinuing them, the options include surgery or endoscopic dilatation for localized disease, or a liquid formula diet,[25] or thiopurine[168] for diffuse disease (Figure 6.1). If patients prove intolerant to azathioprine and/or 6-mercaptopurine, methotrexate[199] or mycophenolate[204] can be tried. Lastly, for the tiny minority (probably about 5%) of patients refractory to or intolerant of all these approaches, and in whom

Table 6.4 Specific treatment of active presentations of Crohn's disease other than ileocaecal Crohn's disease.

Obstructive small bowel disease	Trial of intravenous corticosteroids
	Intravenous fluids and nasogastric suction
	Endoscopic balloon dilatation (if feasible)
	Surgery for non-responders (resection, strictureplasty, division of adhesions)
	Parenteral nutritional support
Intra-abdominal abscess	Broad-spectrum antibiotics
	Percutaneous drainage with localized resection of bowel as necessary
Intestinal fistula	See algorithm in Figure 6.5
Perianal disease	Oral metronidazole/ciprofloxacin (up to 3 months)
	Oral azathioprine or 6-mercaptopurine
	Consider infliximab for non-responders
	Surgery to drain abscesses or insert seton sutures for chronic fistulae
Upper gastrointestinal disease	Corticosteroids
	Proton pump inhibitors for gastroduodenal disease
	Endoscopic balloon dilatation of strictures
	Surgery with strictureplasty (or resection as needed)
Oral disease	Oral, topical or intra-lesional corticosteroids
	Topical tacrolimus or thalidomide
	Referral to specialist in oral medicine

surgery would be inappropriate, for example because of diffuse disease, infliximab is an option, assuming that contra-indications to its use have been excluded.[232,251] How these principles are applied to different clinical scenarios in Crohn's is described below.

Active ileocaecal inflammation

Presentation and investigation

Terminal ileal and ileocaecal Crohn's disease usually presents with pain, diarrhoea and/or a tender mass in the right iliac fossa (Chapter 2). The differential diagnosis includes an appendix mass, caecal carcinoma, lymphoma and ileocaecal tuberculosis, depending on the patient's age and ethnic origin (Chapter 2) (Table 2.12).

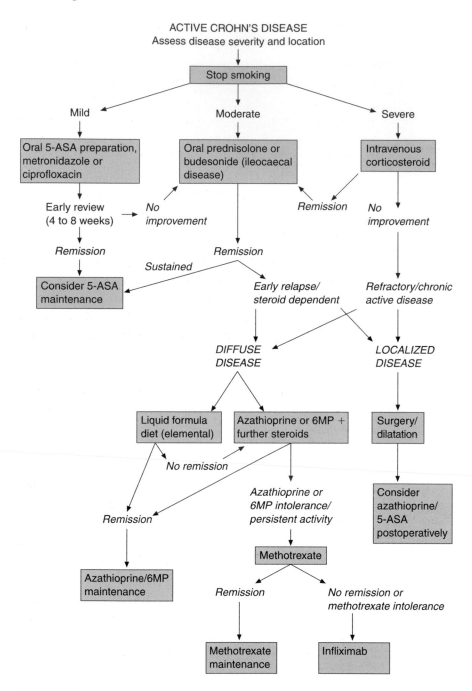

Figure 6.1 *Principles of management of active Crohn's disease. 5-ASA, 5-aminosalicylate; 6MP, 6-mercaptopurine.*

Investigation depends on whether the patient is presenting for the first time or has a relapse of previously diagnosed Crohn's disease. The blood tests shown in Table 6.3 may show evidence of active inflammation and/or undernutrition. A plain abdominal radiograph is essential if intestinal obstruction is suspected. In previously undiagnosed patients, ileo-colonoscopy with biopsy is useful to obtain a tissue diagnosis. Ultrasound and/or CT scan may show thickened, matted bowel loops or an abscess, while barium follow through is useful in defining the extent of disease proximal to the reach of the colonoscope. Radiolabelled leukocyte scans can be helpful to identify sites of bowel inflammation and/or localized collections.

Specific treatment (Figure 6.1)

Aminosalicylates. Patients with mildly or moderately active ileocaecal disease can be tried on high dose oral mesalazine, for example Pentasa 2 g twice daily or Asacol 1.2 g three times daily (Chapter 3).[139,140] Although patients responding to mesalazine tend to be maintained on it long term, there is no evidence that it is effective in maintaining remissions which have been achieved medically.[142]

Antibiotics. Although metronidazole[151] and ciprofloxacin,[159,160] alone or in combination,[154,155,397] are moderately effective in mild to moderately active Crohn's disease (Chapter 3), they are insufficiently potent for use as sole therapy in patients with more severe presentations.

Corticosteroids. In patients with active disease, oral steroids provide the quickest symptomatic response, most patients improving in three to four weeks. Prednisolone (40–60 mg/day) is generally used, the dose being tapered by 5 mg every 7–10 days, once improvement has begun. In patients in whom systemic steroid side-effects are a major problem, budesonide CR (9 mg/day) can be used, albeit at greater cost and with less efficacy.[126] Very sick patients, or those unable to tolerate an oral preparation, need intravenous corticosteroids initially (e.g. hydrocortisone 300–400 mg/day, methyl prednisolone 40–60 mg/day).

In patients on corticosteroids, co-administration of an aminosalicylate confers no additional benefit.[398]

Immunosuppressive drugs. Patients refractory to or dependent on cortico-steroids who, because of extensive disease or previous resection need to avoid surgery, can be treated with adjunctive oral azathioprine (2–2.5 mg/kg per day) or 6-mercaptopurine (1–1.5 mg/kg per day), with the dose of steroids being reduced or phased out as improvement occurs.[119,168] Such patients must be well enough to wait for up to four months for improve-ment. The side-effects of thiopurines make frequent blood counts and liver function tests mandatory (Chapters 3 and 10); to try to reduce the risk of bone marrow suppression, it is also desirable to check TPMT levels or geno-type before initiating therapy (Chapter 3).[164]

Methotrexate given weekly is effective in about 40% of patients not responding to or intolerant of thiopurines (Chapter 3).[195] Mycophenolate mofetil is an alternative of unproven efficacy (Chapter 3).[204] Similarly, ciclosporin is of unproven efficacy in active Crohn's disease (Chapter 3).[212,214,399]

Anti-TNF-α antibody. In patients with persistently active disease despite all the above measures, and in whom surgery is not appropriate, infliximab is a useful new alternative (Figure 6.2) (Chapter 3). Contra-indications are listed in Table 3.10. Current evidence-based recommendations comprise infusions of 5 mg/kg at no more than 14–20-week intervals for up to a year.[231,232,251]

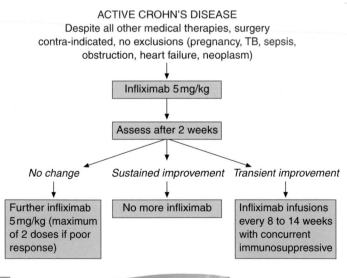

Figure 6.2 *Use of infliximab in Crohn's disease.*

Patients not responding to two infusions are unlikely to improve with further infliximab.[230] Furthermore, patients obtaining a prolonged remission from a single infusion may not need further such therapy. Most authorities recommend concurrent use of immunosuppressive therapy (a thiopurine or methotrexate) to maximize efficacy and minimize delayed hypersensitivity reactions to infliximab (Chapter 3).[191,251]

Dictary therapy. In patients with a poor response to or preference for avoiding corticosteroids, in those with extensive small bowel disease and in children (Chapter 8), an alternative primary therapy is a liquid formula diet (Chapter 5). Liquid diets given for four to six weeks as the sole nutritional source approach corticosteroids in efficacy,[25,26] but there is a high relapse rate on resumption of a normal diet.

Surgery. In patients whose ileocaecal disease fails to respond to drug or dietary therapy, particularly if they have short-segment (less than 20 cm) rather than extensive disease, surgery is indicated (Chapter 4).

Patients at particular risk of responding poorly to medical therapy include those with stenotic disease, extraintestinal manifestations and a history of more than five years' duration.[400] Furthermore, some patients prefer surgery at presentation to the prospect of pharmacological or nutritional treatment of uncertain duration and safety; however, there are as yet no controlled data to confirm which approach is best.[401,402]

Obstructive small bowel Crohn's disease

Presentation and investigation

In patients presenting with obstructive symptoms and signs, with appropriate abnormalities on plain abdominal radiograph, it is important to decide whether stricturing results from active inflammation, fibrosis with scarring or adhesions caused by previous surgery. Laboratory markers and/or radiolabelled leukocyte scan can help to identify individuals with active inflammatory Crohn's disease. An abdominal CT scan gives further useful information about the site of disease and pathology underlying this presentation, but small bowel barium studies may exacerbate the symptoms in patients who are obstructed.

Specific treatment (Table 6.4)

In most patients, a short trial of intravenous corticosteroids is given in addition to intravenous fluids and, if necessary, nasogastric suction. If this treatment is successful, treatment continues as for severe inflammatory Crohn's disease (see above). Patients responding to conservative therapy should be given a low residue diet to reduce the chance of recurrent symptoms.

In patients not settling after 48–72 hours of conservative treatment, surgery is needed, options being local resection, strictureplasty or endoscopic balloon dilatation (Figure 6.3) (Chapter 4). In patients presenting with obstructive symptoms who are not likely to resume an oral diet in less than five to seven days, parenteral nutrition is recommended.

Intra-abdominal abscess

Ultrasound, CT scan and/or radiolabelled leukocyte scan are used to confirm suspected intra-abdominal abscess in patients with Crohn's. Broad-spectrum antibiotics are given and the abscess drained either percutaneously under radiological control or surgically. Subsequent treatment is of the underlying pathological process, for example ileocaecal inflammation with fistulation.

Intestinal fistulae

Investigation

The relevant anatomical connections are clarified using contrast radiology (Figure 6.4), CT scan, endoluminal ultrasound and/or MRI (Chapter 2). In

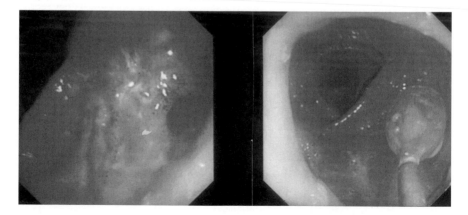

Figure 6.3 *Colonoscopic balloon dilation of an anastomotic stricture in Crohn's disease. (a) Narrowed ileocolonic anastomosis and (b) through-the-endoscope balloon inserted into the stricture and dilated.*

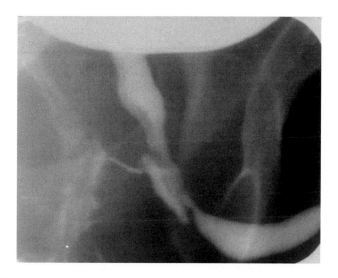

Figure 6.4 *Micturating cystogram showing recto-urethral fistula in Crohn's disease. The fistula can be seen between the rectum (left) and urethra (centre).*

patients with high-output enterocutaneous fistulae, electrolyte and fluid balance and nutritional status also require careful evaluation (Chapter 9).

Specific treatment (Figure 6.5)
Restitution of nutritional well-being is required using enteral or parenteral nutrition, depending on the site and output of the fistula. Uncontrolled evidence suggests that medical therapy with oral, rectal or intravenous metronidazole, ciprofloxacin and/or a thiopurine[168] causes some fistulae to heal. Infliximab is an option in some patients,[115,232,233,251] but its long-term efficacy and safety are not yet clear (Chapter 3).

Fistulae which fail to heal after a few weeks need surgical intervention (Chapter 4). Risk factors include the presence of distal obstruction, the fistula arising from a grossly diseased segment of bowel and a short tract between the skin and bowel.[403]

Active Crohn's colitis
Management of Crohn's colitis usually resembles that for active ileocaecal disease (Table 6.5).

High doses of aminosalicylates (Pentasa 2 g bd or Asacol 1.2 g tds) may be effective in patients with mildly active Crohn's colitis. Furthermore, metronidazole (400 mg bd for up to three months) is of greater benefit in colonic than

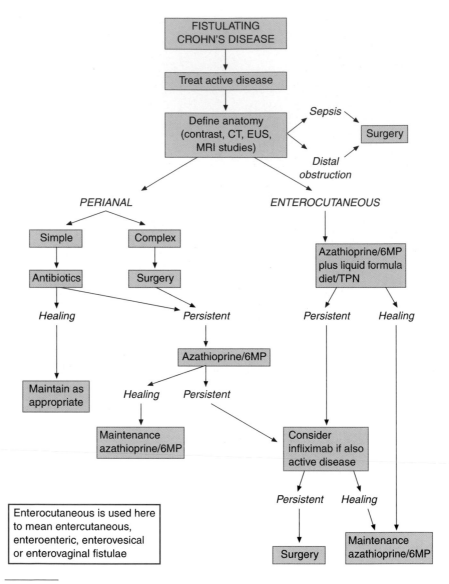

Figure 6.5 *Treatment of fistulizing Crohn's disease. CT, computerized tomography; MRI, magnetic resonance imaging; EUS, endoscopic ultrasound; 6MP, 6-mercaptopurine; TPN, total parenteral nutrition.*

ileal Crohn's disease, with a response rate of about 50%.[151] Limited meta-analysis data suggest that Crohn's colitis responds to a liquid formula diet.[26]

Patients with more severe attacks require corticosteroids orally and sometimes intravenously, with the addition of a thiopurine or methotrexate if

Table 6.5 Specific treatment of active Crohn's colitis.[312]

Drug therapy	Corticosteroids intravenously (hydrocortisone or methylprednisolone) then oral prednisolone
	High dose 5-ASA orally
	Metronidazole orally for mild disease
	Azathioprine or 6-mercaptopurine (if response can be postponed <4 months)
	Methotrexate (for azathioprine/6-mercaptopurine refractory or intolerant patients)
	Infliximab (for patients refractory to or intolerant of all of the above)
Nutritional therapy	Liquid formula diet
Endoscopic therapy	Balloon dilatation of strictures
Surgery	Total colectomy with ileostomy (pouch usually contra-indicated)
	Segmental resection for localized stricture

their disease flares on dose-tapering. Infliximab is an option in patients non-responsive to or intolerant of the above therapies. About 70% of patients with total Crohn's colitis come to surgery eventually (Chapter 4).[68]

Active perianal disease

Presentation and investigation
Perianal involvement is common in Crohn's and management is summarized in Table 6.4. Its investigation is outlined in Chapter 4.

Treatment of perianal abscesses and fistulae
Perianal or perirectal abscesses require surgical drainage, often with insertion of a long-term seton suture (Chapter 4). Thereafter, medical treatment of the associated fistulation is necessary (see below). Non-suppurative perianal complications of Crohn's disease may benefit from careful local hygiene including the use of sitz baths.

Uncontrolled trials suggest that metronidazole alone,[156] or in combination with ciprofloxacin[349] heals about 50% of perianal fistulae, although recurrence on cessation of therapy is common.[404] Injection of a fibrin sealant may close some fistulae.[405]

Prospective[114] and retrospective reports[406] suggested that 6-mercaptopurine (1.5 mg/kg per day) is beneficial in patients with perianal disease, although a recent meta-analysis has failed to confirm a statistically significant benefit for the thiopurines.[168]

An alternative immunosuppressive treatment not tested in controlled trials is intravenous ciclosporin with or without a subsequent thiopurine.[215,407] In a recent placebo-controlled trial oral tacrolimus (0.2 mg/kg per day) improved fistula output by 43% compared with 8% in placebo-controlled patients; unfortunately only 10% of patients on tacrolimus had complete fistula closure.[220]

Although infliximab has been shown in controlled trials to heal some perianal fistulae,[115,233] reopening of tracts is common after its discontinuation (Chapter 3). Indeed, the cost of treatment of uncomplicated perianal fistulae with infliximab is difficult to justify since the outcome in terms of healing at one year with infliximab is not significantly better than when metronidazole and/or thiopurines are used.[232,235]

Upper gastrointestinal Crohn's disease

The rarity of symptomatic upper gastrointestinal Crohn's disease precludes a controlled evidence base for its treatment; suggested management is outlined in Table 6.4.

It has been claimed that acid suppression with proton pump inhibitors is effective in Crohn's disease affecting the oesophagus, stomach and duodenum,[409,410] and corticosteroids and immunosuppressive agents are used as for Crohn's affecting other sites in the gut.[60,61] Endoscopic balloon dilatation of short strictures can be attempted;[335] formal surgical approaches are discussed in Chapter 4.

Oral Crohn's disease

Patients with oral Crohn's disease are best managed in close conjunction with specialists in oral medicine. However, there are no controlled data to guide treatment of oral Crohn's disease. Topical and intralesional steroids help some patients.[411] Topical tacrolimus[222] and oral thalidomide[259] are new alternatives, although the side-effects of the latter preclude its widespread use (Chapter 3). Case reports indicate possible efficacy for infliximab.[412]

Some reports suggest a pathogenic role for cinnamon aldehyde, cocoa, curry agents and synthetic preservatives such as benzoate, but the value of diets excluding these and other food components needs confirmation in controlled studies.

Maintenance of remission in Crohn's disease

Stopping smoking

The most effective prophylactic measure in patients who smoke is to stop: the risk of relapse in non-smokers at 5 years is reduced by about 40%.[22,23] Furthermore, stopping smoking improves the natural history of Crohn's disease, particularly in women.[24]

Drug prophylaxis

The efficacy of drug prophylaxis depends on whether remission has been achieved by medical or surgical treatment (Table 6.6).

Patients in remission after medical treatment

Aminosalicylates. Meta-analysis shows that, unlike in UC, long-term aminosalicylates have little or no prophylactic effect in patients whose remission has been achieved by medical therapy.[142]

Corticosteroids. Prednisolone has no prophylactic role.[413] Unfortunately, budesonide CR (6 mg/day), which is less likely to cause steroid-related complications such as osteoporosis, does not reduce relapse rate at one year, although it does prolong the time to relapse after medically achieved remission.[131,132]

Thiopurines. In corticosteroid-dependent patients, azathioprine (2–2.5 mg/kg per day) and 6-mercaptopurine (1–1.5 mg/kg per day) are of proven value in maintaining remission and reducing steroid requirements.[168] Treatment should be continued for four to five years in the first instance (Chapter 3).[170]

Table 6.6 Maintenance of remission in Crohn's disease.[312]

All patients	Stop smoking
Remission achieved medically	No standard treatment of proven value
	Azathioprine/6-mercaptopurine or
	methotrexate for refractory disease
	Fish oil (Purepa) possibly
Remission achieved surgically	Aminosalicylates (for ileal disease)
	Metronidazole (3 months only)
	Azathioprine or 6-mercaptopurine

Methotrexate. Weekly intramuscular methotrexate (15 mg/week) in patients not responding to or intolerant of thiopurines is superior to placebo in maintaining remission of Crohn's.[199] Controlled data do not exist for the use of oral methotrexate or for its use for more than a year (Chapter 3). Nevertheless, anecdotal experience suggests that oral methotrexate (15–25 mg/week) can be used safely and effectively for at least two years in thiopurine-failing patients.

Ciclosporin. There is no evidence to support the use of ciclosporin for maintenance of remission in Crohn's disease.[214,399]

Infliximab. In patients with very refractory disease, infliximab can be used to induce and then maintain remission and minimize steroid use.[230,231,251] However, existing data do not extend beyond a year and its costs and possible side-effects mean that such therapy cannot yet be justified for use for more prolonged periods (Chapter 3).

Fish oil. High-potency ileal-release fish oil capsules (Purepa), if commercially available, would be an attractive option should their prophylactic efficacy in one study be confirmed (Chapter 3).[300]

Patients in remission after surgical treatment (Figure 6.6)
About half of patients undergoing resection for ileocaecal Crohn's disease have a clinical relapse within five years and half will need a second operation by ten years.[414] Unfortunately, there are few data to support the use of drugs to reduce the rate of symptomatic as opposed to endoscopic postoperative recurrence in patients with Crohn's disease.[82]

Aminosalicylates. A meta-analysis[142] covering four trials[415–418] suggested that long-term aminosalicylates slightly reduced the risk of symptomatic relapse after surgery: a risk reduction of 13% meant that the number of patients needing to be treated (NNT) to prevent one recurrence was eight. However, a more recent placebo-controlled European study[143] showed no advantage for Pentasa (4 g/day) except in patients with localized ileal disease, in whom clinical relapse rate at 18 months was 22% on Pentasa and 40% on placebo. Reassessment thereafter of the data analysed in Cammá's meta-analysis[142] after inclusion of the European results[143] and exclusion of Caprilli's trial,[415] which was not blinded or placebo-controlled, dropped the risk reduction to

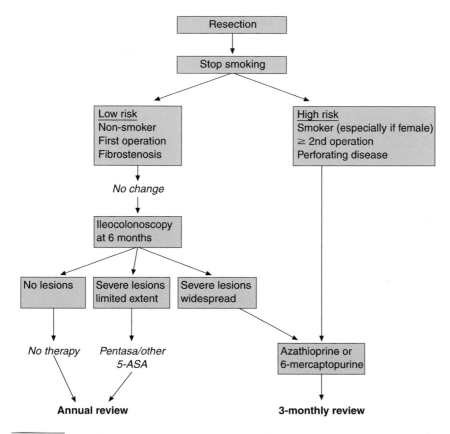

Figure 6.6 *Empirical approach to prophylaxis after resection for ileocaecal Crohn's disease. (Reproduced from Rutgeerts. Gut 2002; **11**: 152–3[423] with permission from the BMJ Publishing Group.)*

only 8% (NNT 12).[144,145] This NNT is probably too high to support use of aminosalicylates for postoperative prophylaxis except in the minority of patients with exclusively ileal disease.

Nitroimidazole antibiotics. Oral metronidazole (400 mg tds for three months only) reduced symptomatic as well as endoscopic recurrence one year after surgery, but the clinical advantage over placebo was lost beyond that period.[157] Unfortunately, although also efficacious in reducing clinical and endoscopic relapse one year after surgery, another nitroimidazole, ornidazole (1 g/day for a year), was no better tolerated than metronidazole and cannot therefore be recommended for routine postoperative prophylaxis.[419]

Budesonide. Controlled ileal release budesonide (6 mg/day) halved the postoperative endoscopic recurrence rate at one year for inflammatory but not fibrostenotic Crohn's, but clinical relapses were as common as in placebo-treated patients.[420]

Thiopurines. In a controlled study in children, 6-mercaptopurine was more effective in preventing postoperative relapse over a two-year period than 5-ASA drugs or no medication.[421] Similarly, low dose 6-mercaptopurine (50 mg/day) was better than placebo and aminosalicylates in preventing symptomatic, endoscopic and radiological recurrence after surgery in adults.[189] However, the placebo relapse rate was 70% at two years and a recurrence rate of 53% for patients given 6-mercaptopurine scarcely represents a ringing endorsement of this treatment, particularly in view of its potential side-effects. Thiopurines need further evaluation, at full dose, for postoperative prophylaxis.

Other options. Interleukin-10 was no better than placebo in preventing postoperative endoscopic or clinical relapse at one year in a recent study;[291] neither was the probiotic *Lactobacillus GG*.[422] Trials of other biological therapies including infliximab, of antibiotics and probiotics, fish oil,[300] a liquid formula diet and other immunomodulatory approaches would be of interest.

Conclusions

Apart from stopping smoking, no therapeutic measure can be unreservedly recommended for routine prophylaxis after ileal resection for Crohn's. Although colonoscopy at, say, six months after surgery might be used to select patients, according to the severity of endoscopic recurrence,[82] for specific therapies, the validity of this approach needs confirmation in further clinical trials.

So what should surgeons and physicians recommend? They should urge smokers to stop (Figure 6.6). A discussion with the immediately postoperative patient about the available pharmacological evidence is often concluded by patients with uncomplicated disease indicating their enthusiasm to be off all tablets after months or years of such treatment. Patients with exclusively ileal disease can be advised, however, to use Pentasa (4 g/day).[143] It is reasonable to suggest that those with aggressive, perforating or extensive disease, or a second or later resection, take a thiopurine in full dose, despite the lack of data to support this approach.

chapter 7

Crohn's disease in relation to sexuality and pregnancy

Introduction

Crohn's disease and its treatment carries special implications for women of childbearing age. In this chapter, management aspects of the influence of Crohn's disease on sexuality, fertility, pregnancy, breast-feeding and the prognosis thereafter are considered.

Psychosexual factors

Many patients have problems with their body image, self-confidence and sexual relationships as a result of their disease, particularly if they have a stoma or perianal disease.[113] Patients with stomas tend to fear intimate relationships.[113] Indeed, the partners of patients with stomas are likely to be more accepting than the patient themselves.[424] Counselling of both partners before and after the formation of a stoma is therefore essential. Patients may also experience problems with the appearance-modifying effects of corticosteroids.[113]

Women with Crohn's disease have a high incidence of dyspareunia and vaginal discharge (60%); they more often have infrequent or no intercourse (24%) than women in the general population (4%).[425,426] In men, the risk of impotence is highest after proctocolectomy (4–8%).[427]

Despite these figures, most patients appear satisfied with their sexual function.[424] Many, however, will not necessarily volunteer their problems in a busy outpatient clinic, and the opportunity to visit a psychosexual counsellor can be invaluable.

Oral contraceptive pill

The prevalence of Crohn's disease among users of the oral contraceptive pill (OCP) is increased, the relative risk compared to non-users being about two-fold and returning to normal when the pill is stopped.[38,428] The OCP may also cause a segmental colitis resembling Crohn's, except that it resolves on withdrawing the drug.[429] The current consensus, however, is that the modern low-dose OCP is safe in non-smoking patients with IBD and that its use is preferable to unwanted pregnancy.[428]

Inheritance

Relatives of patients with Crohn's disease are at increased risk of IBD (Chapter 1). Useful figures to quote to potential parents are that the overall risk of a child developing Crohn's is about 10% if one parent has either type of IBD and up to 40% if both parents do.[430]

Fertility

Women

Fertility is normal in patients with quiescent Crohn's, but reduced in those with active disease.[431] The reasons for reduced fertility in active Crohn's may include dyspareunia, particularly in the presence of severe perianal disease, impaired ovulation or fallopian tube blockage as a result of pelvic sepsis, hormonal changes, treatment for Crohn's (see below) and/or avoiding pregnancy on well-meaning but sometimes misguided medical advice. In the latter context, in one study, 25% of women were advised by doctors to avoid having a family.[432] This may explain why fewer pregnancies occur in patients in whom the diagnosis of IBD was made before rather than after their first pregnancy.[433]

Men

Little information exists about male fertility and IBD, although the number of pregnancies resulting from men with Crohn's disease is reduced compared with the general population.[434] Impaired libido and oligospermia occur in patients with active disease.[435]

The biggest risk to fertility in men is treatment with sulphasalazine, which causes reversible abnormalities in sperm number and function in about 60%

of patients.[436] The sulphonamide moiety causes this effect, which is reversible on stopping sulphasalazine or switching to an alternative amino-salicylate. Thiopurines have no effect on the quality of semen in patients with Crohn's.[183]

Pregnancy

Effect of pregnancy on Crohn's disease

The yearly relapse rate in pregnant patients with Crohn's resembles that in non-pregnant patients.[437,438] However, if Crohn's is active at the time of conception, it is likely to remain active or even worsen, so that aggressive therapy is indicated (see below).[439]

Effect of Crohn's disease on outcome of pregnancy

In one study of nearly 750 pregnancies, 83% of patients with Crohn's had healthy offspring, 12% spontaneous abortion, 2% stillbirth and 1% a child with congenital abnormality.[439] In patients becoming pregnant during remission and remaining in remission throughout pregnancy, the likelihood of spontaneous abortion, stillbirth and congenital abnormality resembles that in the general population.[440] However, in patients with active disease at conception, or who relapse during pregnancy, stillbirth and preterm delivery are all more likely. Other factors adversely affecting the outcome of pregnancy in patients with Crohn's include ileal involvement, previous bowel resection and smoking.[438,441]

Effect of nutrition on outcome of pregnancy

Poor maternal nutrition adversely affects the fetus, so that nutritional supplementation including folate should be given as necessary. A liquid formula diet has been used successfully in active small bowel Crohn's in pregnancy.[696]

Investigation of IBD in pregnancy

Blood tests may be difficult to interpret in pregnancy since falls in haemoglobin and albumin concentrations, a fall in platelet count and a rise in ESR and alkaline phosphatase (of placental origin) are physiological.[442] Upper and lower GI endoscopy appear to be safe[443] as is ultrasound. Radiation should be avoided as far as possible. A plain abdominal radiograph may be necessary if perforation, obstruction or toxic megacolon are suspected, but contrast radiology and CT scans are contra-indicated because of the risk of fetal damage.

Effects of drugs used in treatment of IBD on pregnancy (Table 7.1)

Aminosalicylates

Sulphasalazine and the newer aminosalicylates are safe in pregnancy for mother and fetus.[444-446]

Corticosteroids

Corticosteroids do not appear to be teratogenic; other fetal side-effects such as adrenal suppression are rare.[446] Any risks associated with use of corticosteroids in pregnancy are clearly outweighed by the greater risks to both mother and fetus of undertreatment of active Crohn's.

Antibiotics

Metronidazole given for treatment of trichomonas in pregnancy appears not to affect the fetus,[447] but it may not be safe to use this drug for the longer periods needed for treatment of Crohn's (Chapters 3 and 6).[448] Although use of ciprofloxacin in pregnancy is not advised because of the risk of birth defects, a recent prospective trial showed no increase in fetal abnormalities with this drug.[449]

Thiopurines

Retrospective studies have shown no increase in adverse outcomes of pregnancy in IBD patients given thiopurines.[179,180] Discussion of the possible risks

Table 7.1 Safety in pregnancy of drugs used to treat Crohn's disease.

Safe	Contra-indicated
5-Aminosalicylates	Metronidazole (more than 1 week)
Corticosteroids	Ciprofloxacin
Metronidazole (for up to 1 week)	Ciclosporin
Thiopurines	Methotrexate
	Mycophenolate
	Infliximab
	Thalidomide

with the patient and her partner is recommended, but if thiopurines are necessary to maintain remission in a patient with IBD, it is reasonable on current evidence to continue with this treatment. However, because of the potential early side-effects associated with the initiation of thiopurine therapy (Chapter 3), these drugs should not be started for the first time in pregnant patients.[216] Thiopurines taken by men at the time of fertilization may slightly increase the risk of spontaneous abortion and congenital abnormalities.[183]

Other immunosuppressive and immunomodulatory drugs

Although ciclosporin has been used apparently safely in pregnant patients with acute severe UC, the limited evidence base for its prescription in Crohn's disease (Chapter 3) makes it hard to justify the risks of hypertension and nephrotoxicity in pregnant patients with this type of IBD. Methotrexate is abortifacient, mutagenic and teratogenic and is contra-indicated in pregnancy.[448] Both men and women should avoid conception when taking and within six months of stopping methotrexate.[194,448] Mycophenolate is teratogenic and should not be prescribed in pregnancy. Neither infliximab nor thalidomide should be used in pregnancy because of the risk of fetal damage,[259,450] but limited data about the outcome of inadvertent pregnancies in patients on infliximab have been reassuring.[248]

Effect of surgery for IBD on pregnancy

Surgery during pregnancy should be restricted to patients with urgent indications such as obstruction unresponsive to medical therapy, perforation, massive haemorrhage or toxic megacolon.[432] For acute colonic manifestations, total colectomy with exteriorization of the resection margins has been suggested to optimize outcome prior to definitive surgery after delivery.[451] Although total colectomy carries a 60% risk of spontaneous abortion,[216] prompt surgical intervention where essential is thought to improve maternal and fetal outcome.[451]

Childbirth

The rate of caesarean section is slightly higher (about 20%) in patients with Crohn's than in the general population (15%).[452] Although vaginal delivery reproducibly worsens symptoms in patients with active perianal disease,[452] a similar deterioration may occur even after caesarean section.[453]

Patients without major colonic or perianal disease can usually have a vaginal delivery safely even in the presence of a stoma, although the latter may prolapse during pregnancy. Episiotomy should be avoided since it predisposes to perianal involvement in Crohn's, even in patients with none before the procedure.[454]

Breast-feeding

Despite concerns that the sulphonamide component of sulphasalazine might cause kernicterus after transmission to the newborn child through breast milk, its binding site to albumin is different from that for bilirubin and neonatal jaundice is not a particular problem.[455] 5-ASA is poorly absorbed from the gut and little appears in breast milk: no adverse affects have been reported in breast-fed infants.[456]

Prednisolone taken by the mother is also poorly concentrated in breast milk and appears to be safe.[457]

Azathioprine and 6-mercaptopurine have been used safely during breast-feeding of the children of mothers with renal transplants and systemic lupus erythematosis,[458] but this practice is not recommended by the manufacturers. As with the use of thiopurines in pregnancy, an informed discussion with the patient and her partner is advisable. There are no data on the safety of breast-feeding by mothers with Crohn's disease taking other immunosuppressive agents.

Long-term outcome of Crohn's disease after pregnancy

Parity in women with Crohn's appears to improve the long-term outcome of the disease. In one study, well-nourished patients had fewer relapses of their disease in the three years after a pregnancy than in the three years leading up to it.[437] Furthermore, in patients with ileocolonic Crohn's, the number of resections over a 10–15-year follow-up was fewer in those who had been pregnant before diagnosis than in non-parous women. The interval from first to subsequent resection was also longer in parous patients.[459] Possible mechanisms of the apparently protective effect of pregnancy include reduced immune responsiveness and/or delayed fibrous stricture formation, as a result of pregnancy.

chapter 8

Management of Crohn's disease in children

Epidemiology

Between June 1998 and July 1999 it was estimated that 5.2/100 000 children of less than 16 years of age in the UK and Republic of Ireland were affected by IBD.[460] This prospective study surveyed over 3000 paediatricians, adult and paediatric gastroenterologists, paediatric surgeons and pathologists utilizing the resources of the British Paediatric Surveillance Unit and British Society of Gastroenterology. It is planned to repeat this study soon to see if, as has been suggested by retrospective studies, the incidence of Crohn's disease in children is increasing.[461] Unlike adults, the majority of these children with IBD had Crohn's disease (60%), with ulcerative colitis (28%) and indeterminate colitis (12%) making up the remainder.

Crohn's disease in children compared with adults

In addition to having the condition for a longer part of their lives, there is evidence that the disease per se is more severe.

Growth and pubertal delay, which occur in up to 35% of subjects,[462] are complications specific to the younger age group and are issues not dealt with in adult units. The aetiology of this growth failure remains controversial. Historically, it was thought to be a consequence of reduced nutrition. More recent clinical and laboratory data indicate that the growth suppression could be due to the effects of cytokines, such as interleukin-6, associated with chronic inflammation (Chapter 1), and that it is vital to keep the disease under control in order to maximize growth and pubertal development.[462,463]

Crohn's disease may have an even greater psychosocial impact in children, and their families, than it does in adults; this topic is discussed in Chapter 9.

Clinical assessment and investigation

Assessment of children includes evaluation of their symptoms, nutrition, growth and pubertal data, acute phase reactants and endoscopic and histological status.

Imaging

Diagnosis of Crohn's disease requires total colonoscopy, barium follow-through and upper endoscopy (see Chapter 2). The latter has revealed a high incidence of inflammation in the stomach and duodenum.[464]

Radiolabelled leukocyte scans are not routinely used in most paediatric gastroenterology centres, one reason being the risk of false-positive and false-negative scans (Chapter 2).[465]

Auxology

Accurate auxological measurements, including pubertal staging,[466] are essential to the management of children with Crohn's disease. Recording of children's height and weight is often poor.[467] Impaired height is more common at diagnosis in Crohn's disease than in UC (13% vs 3%) and growth failure has been detected both before the development of intestinal symptoms[468] and during relapses.[469]

Activity indices and quality of life assessment

As in adults, a variety of scoring systems are available to assess disease activity, although these are largely used for research. One score validated in children is the paediatric Crohn's disease activity index (PCDAI) which includes subjective and objective measures.[470] Others include the Crohn's disease activity index modified for children. In practice, most paediatric gastroenterologists rely on their overall assessment of the patient. A more formalized version of this (physician global assessment) has been shown to correlate well with the PCDAI.[471]

To assess quality of life issues, now a key component of clinically based research and the development of new drugs, a quality of life index has been developed for children with IBD;[472] this has been adapted and validated for use in UK children.[473]

Principles of treatment

The aims of treatment in children with Crohn's disease are to induce and then maintain clinical remission. It is vital also to maximize growth and pubertal development for the future.

As in adults, management of Crohn's disease in children is best organized by experienced multi-disciplinary departments; these include, in addition to paediatric gastroenterologists, child psychologists or psychiatrists, dietitians and paediatric surgeons. Smooth handover to the adult services is essential; the age at which this is most appropriate depends on the maturity and knowledge of the children and their families. In our unit, transfer to adult gastroenterologists with a special interest in IBD occurs in joint clinics when patients have completed growth and pubertal development at the age of 16–18 years.

Treatment options

Evidence base

Treatments used in children are similar to those used in adults. The main difference is the widespread use in children of enteral nutrition (EN) for inducing remission to avoid the growth-suppressing effects of corticosteroids.

The author (NMC) is a member of the British Society of Paediatric Gastroenterology, Hepatology and Nutrition IBD Working Group writing evidence-based guidelines for drug and nutritional treatment of paediatric IBD (due to be completed 2003) (http://www.bspghan.org.uk). Using the criteria of the Scottish Intercollegiate Guidelines Network (SIGN), the working group has concluded that there are almost no well-designed or satisfactorily conducted, randomized, controlled trials of treatments of Crohn's disease in children.

In particular, the evidence for all drugs other than corticosteroids and enteral nutrition is based mainly on controlled studies performed in adults and on small observational studies in children. Reasons for this include, historically, a reluctance to undertake research in children for ethical reasons and difficulties in recruiting sufficient numbers for trials. Furthermore, the relatively small numbers of children with Crohn's disease reduce the financial motivation for the pharmaceutical industry to fund clinical trials.

Enteral nutrition

In the UK, the most commonly used treatment for Crohn's disease is enteral nutrition (EN) involving a six to eight week course of an exclusive polymeric or elemental enteral feed (e.g. Modulin-IBD, Nestle, UK or EO28, SHS) (Chapter 5). A lack of appropriate trials means that the long term benefits of EN as the treatment of choice of Crohn's disease in children remain uncertain. What is clear is that enteral feeds are as effective as steroids in attaining remission and have the advantage of avoiding steroid-related side-effects such as growth suppression.

Enteral nutrition for induction of remission

Use of EN was first reported in adults in 1977[474] and in children in 1981.[475] In 1983, O'Morain described 15 children who responded to an elemental diet with improvement in linear growth in three of the group.[476] In a randomized study using a semi-elemental feed, EN was as efficacious as steroids and gave better short term growth (measured over 6 months).[477] Others have confirmed these data for elemental diets.[478,479]

Polymeric diets, which are cheaper and more palatable, have also been found to be as effective as steroids.[480] During treatment with polymeric EN around 80% of children show a good clinical response.[385,463] Reduction of both serum and mucosal inflammatory cytokine levels has been demonstrated.[385,481] In the latter study, decreases of ESR and IL-6 occurred as early as three days after commencing enteral diet. These were followed at day 7 by decreases in PCDAI and in serum C-reactive protein concentration and an increase in circulating levels of insulin-like growth factor (IGF-I). In contrast, none of the nutritional variables assessed, such as weight for age and mid-upper arm circumference, changed significantly until day 14.[481] These results indicate that polymeric diets act primarily by reducing inflammation rather than improving nutrition.

Supplementation of feeds with glutamine has been proposed to be of benefit in catabolic patients. A randomized, blinded study in 18 children with Crohn's, however, failed to demonstrate any significant benefit of glutamine supplementation.[377]

A meta-analysis of EN in the treatment of active Crohn's disease in children examined five randomized trials with a total of 147 patients, the largest including 68 patients, and found that EN was as effective as steroids at inducing remission.[482] Another 12 non-randomized studies were identified and excluded from the meta-analysis. The authors estimated that an additional 10 randomized studies with results similar to the largest study to date would be required to demonstrate a benefit of steroids over EN. While most effective in children with primarily small bowel disease, EN can also be used for those with colonic disease.

Mechanism of action of enteral nutrition

The mechanism of action of EN is much debated (Chapter 5). Possibilities include alteration of the intestinal bacterial milieu, anti-inflammatory constituents of the feeds (for example the cytokine transforming growth factor beta (TGF-β) which is present in Modulin-IBD[385]) or the limited protein exposure in the feeds used.[483] Understanding how EN works may help explain the pathogenesis of Crohn's disease and give clues for further treatment options.

Enteral nutrition for the maintenance of remission

The rate of relapse in long-term studies following EN has not been clarified. A recent abstract has suggested that enteral feeds delay the use of steroids by only about 19 weeks.[484] We recently reported the results of using EN to treat 36 children newly diagnosed with Crohn's disease over a two-year period. 80% went into remission using EN alone, the remainder requiring steroids. After a median follow up of 1.25 years, 54% had relapsed and 46% remained in remission; overall 58% were managed solely with enteral feeds and 5-ASA compounds.[485] In Bristol, of 44 children followed up for three years, 47% had completely avoided steroids and steroid use was delayed by 68 weeks.[486] Longer follow-up is required to establish the role of EN and steroids for long-term management of Crohn's disease.

In a controlled trial, Belli and coworkers reported the use of an elemental feed given by overnight nasogastric tube for one in every four months to children with Crohn's disease and growth failure.[487] In the treatment group, growth failure was reversed and steroid use and CDAI reduced. A similar outcome was reported by a second group.[488] In a retrospective study, Wilchanski et al found that children continuing on nasogastric feeds had a prolonged time to relapse and improved linear growth.[489] Whether similar results can be achieved with daytime oral supplementation in patients in clinical remission has not been established, although such an approach is already commonly adopted.

Practicalities of enteral feeding

The main disadvantage of EN is that patients find it difficult to take the feed exclusively for a prolonged period. In our unit, a consistent and positive message to children, parents, nursing staff and junior doctors leads to a high level of compliance with good clinical outcomes. This is in part because patients see their peers getting better.

New patients are established on EN as inpatients for two to three days and are then reviewed at one to two weekly intervals to monitor clinical status and weight and to encourage compliance. The majority feel considerably better within one week of starting the treatment; if not responding by two weeks, they usually need other therapy such as steroids or surgery for strictures. Patients who have had EN before can often be managed at home during relapse, although they may respond better if very unwell when admitted to hospital for a few days. The majority of patients take the feed orally although some require nasogastric tubes. For those requiring frequent courses percutaneous gastrostomies have been used safely.[490]

The type of feed does not appear to be critical. Elemental, semi-elemental and polymeric feeds have all been successful and the choice will largely depend on the local unit.

The period of enteral feeding for patients with active Crohn's disease is also not uniform. In our unit, a six-week course of a polymeric formula is given either orally or by nasogastric tube; others use an eight-week course.[385] Modulin-IBD is approximately 1 calorie/ml and the total calories given equal the daily estimated average requirements for the patient's age. At the end of the course of EN, individual foods are introduced over the subsequent four to six weeks depending on the response of the individual patient; over the same period the quantity of EN is gradually reduced. We have found that the largest reduction in PCDAI in children treated with EN was at four weeks; whether reintroducing foods at this stage would lead to an increased risk of relapse needs to be clarified.[463]

Complications of enteral feeding

Complications of enteral feeding are unusual. Some children may be allergic to the protein in polymeric feeds. These children get much worse diarrhoea during the feed and changing to an elemental formula can resolve the problem. The lack of dietary fibre during EN can lead to constipation, particularly two to three months after completing the course. This may present as abdominal pain (without any associated rise in inflammatory markers); it is essential to remember constipation as a possible cause of pain before considering other treatments for disease relapse.

Corticosteroids

Efficacy

A reducing course of prednisolone (1–2 mg/kg per day up to 60 mg), the most commonly used steroid in the UK, is effective in inducing remission in most children with active Crohn's disease. Alternate day prednisolone is often used once children have clinically improved and are on lower doses, with the aim of reducing steroid-related growth suppression.[491]

In adults, meta-analyses[25,26] and the Cochrane Library Systematic Review[492] suggest that steroids are more efficacious than enteral feeds for the treatment of acute Crohn's disease (Chapter 5). However, as indicated above, in paediatric studies enteral feeds appear to be as efficacious as steroids.[482] Possible explanations for this difference are better compliance, a higher proportion of newly diagnosed patients and a longer course of enteral nutrition used in paediatric studies.

There are few studies of budesonide (Chapter 3) in the paediatric population. In an uncontrolled study of children with ileocaecal Crohn's disease, about 60% responded but linear growth did not improve.[493] A retrospective study reported that the efficacy of budesonide was less than of prednisolone, although better than mesalazine.[494] A multi-centre, double-blind, placebo-controlled European trial showed that budesonide was less effective (remission rate of 55% versus 71%) but caused fewer side-effects (moon face or acne) than prednisolone.[495] The recruitment rate for the trial was low, partly due to a lengthy list of exclusion criteria.

Side-effects

Of the side-effects of corticosteroids, the risk of growth suppression and bone demineralization are of major importance, particularly in children who may require repeated courses over many years. Compliance is much easier than for EN, although children who have previously had side-effects, such as moon facies, acne or striae, may be reluctant to take further courses.

Cross-sectional studies in children have demonstrated a reduction in bone mineral density (BMD) in more than 40% of children with IBD,[496] the main causes being not only steroid usage[496,497] but also reduced body mass index (BMI).[497] Children with Crohn's disease had lower BMD than those with ulcerative colitis.[497] In our own unit, DEXA scans have demonstrated reduced bone mineral density in up to 66% of children with newly diagnosed IBD, suggesting that osteopenia can be a consequence of the disease rather than the treatments utilized.[498]

Sulphasalazine and 5-ASA preparations

There are no good quality studies in children examining the use of 5-ASA preparations in Crohn's disease and prescribing is again based on adult studies (Chapter 3). In an attempt to study the use of oral slow-release mesalazine in small bowel Crohn's disease, both a preliminary open label and a randomized study were reported in a single article.[499] While there were some indications of benefit with the treatment the design of the study was not strong enough to confirm this.

Sulphasalazine is often preferred in children with associated joint disease despite its higher rate of side-effects than 5-ASA preparations. It is also used in younger children as syrup. Although sulphasalazine is of proven efficacy in children with UC,[500] comparable data for children with Crohn's colitis are not available. Furthermore, there is no evidence to support the widespread practice of using higher doses of sulphasalazine during acute attacks and of prescribing it long term to maintain remission of paediatric Crohn's disease.

Antibiotics

Despite the widespread use of metronidazole and other antibiotics for localized perianal disease with or without abscesses in adults with Crohn's, there is no good evidence base for this practice in children. Prolonged use of metronidazole in one study caused peripheral neuropathy in 11 of 13 patients aged 12 to 22 years; only six were symptomatic.[158] Antibiotics such as ciprofloxacin and metronidazole are also used to induce remission (in combination with steroids) in Crohn's colitis, but again data to support this approach in children are lacking.

Immunomodulation

Azathioprine and 6-mercaptopurine

Azathioprine and its metabolite 6-mercaptopurine (6-MP) are well established treatments for IBD (Chapter 3). As in adults, their main usage in children is as steroid-sparing agents in those with disease which is difficult to control. A double-blinded, randomized, placebo-controlled study of early usage of 6-MP in children with moderate to severe Crohn's disease was shown to reduce the rate of relapse (9% vs 47%) and steroid usage, but there was no difference in linear growth.[501] Whether such results would be obtained in children treated initially with EN rather than prednisolone is not known.

Use of intravenous azathioprine (3 mg/kg per day) in three children with acute fulminant colitis (ulcerative colitis and Crohn's) has been reported, the first of whom had been referred for surgery which the family refused.[502] All three patients were subsequently weaned to oral azathioprine and have remained in remission for over one year. A larger study in adults does not confirm the benefits of intravenous azathioprine (Chapter 3).[166]

Azathioprine takes up to four months to take effect (Chapter 3). Some units are now starting almost all newly diagnosed children with Crohn's disease on an oral thiopurine.[501] Our approach, which is probably the commonest in the UK at present, is to await one or two relapses before initiating azathioprine. How long to continue thiopurine therapy is also not established, the main concern being the theoretical risk of lymphoma for children who may need very prolonged treatment (Chapter 3).

Methotrexate

Methotrexate (Chapter 3) is rarely used in paediatric practice. In an open label study of low dose weekly subcutaneous methotrexate, 14 children who had severe Crohn's disease and had failed to respond to or developed pancreatitis with 6-mercaptopurine were reported as showing some improvement with sustained remission.[503] This option can be considered in patients failing to respond to all other medical treatments and in whom surgery would not be feasible.

Ciclosporin and tacrolimus

Ciclosporin has been used in the treatment of severe, acute Crohn's as well as ulcerative colitis; it may avert or delay the need for surgery, allowing time for patients to become better prepared for this outcome.[504,505] However, a study of newly diagnosed children with Crohn's disease failed to show clinical improvement in those treated with ciclosporin compared with those given conventional treatment.[506]

Oral tacrolimus (FK506) has also been used in the management of steroid resistant severe colitis (ulcerative colitis and Crohn's); of 13 children, nine responded initially and five avoided surgery after one year of follow-up.[507] The absence of controlled data relating to its use and its serious side-effect profile (Chapter 3) means that oral tacrolimus should be considered only in very refractory paediatric Crohn's disease.

Tumour necrosis factor antagonists

Research over the past 10 years has increased our understanding of the role of cytokines in the pathogenesis of inflammatory bowel disease (Chapter 1). TNF-α has been identified as one of the most important pro-inflammatory cytokines[508] and, as in adults, monoclonal antibodies to it can now be used in the treatment of refractory paediatric Crohn's disease (Chapters 3 and 6).

Infliximab

The first, and to date only antibody to TNF-α to be used clinically is infliximab; as described in Chapter 3, this agent has been shown to be effective in inducing both clinical and endoscopic remission.[120] Published evidence for the use of infliximab in children, however, is limited, consisting thus far of retrospective reviews and case reports. Although it does appear to be effective in inducing remission in the short term,[509] there are also few data about its safety in children; one report suggested that delayed systemic reactions are less common in children than adults.[249]

Recently published guidance from National Institute for Clinical Excellence (NICE) recommended that use of infliximab within the NHS in the UK should be restricted to adults with severe, active Crohn's which is refractory to other treatment and for whom surgery is inappropriate.[232] Fistulizing disease alone was not considered to be sufficient justification. These guidelines were not directed at children and indicated that further research and experience was needed in relation to its use in this age group. It is this author's (NMC) opinion that infliximab should be considered before proceeding to surgery, particularly in children who have a high risk of requiring multiple operations over their lifetime.

Thalidomide

Thalidomide, a TNF-α synthesis inhibitor, was reported to be effective in four out of five boys with Crohn's disease unresponsive to standard therapies.[510] The fifth developed symptoms of a peripheral neuropathy but had normal nerve conduction studies. As indicated in Chapter 3, novel small molecular weight TNF antagonists are under development and are likely in due course to supercede thalidomide as a therapeutic option in children as well as adults.

Topical treatments

Where Crohn's disease is localized to the anus, rectum and distal colon, topical treatments such as steroid and mesalazine enemas can be used to control the symptoms. Formal evidence to support this approach in children, however, is lacking, as it is in adults.

Topical tacrolimus has also been used successfully for treating both oral and perianal Crohn's disease,[222] but systemic absorption[511] may lead to serious side-effects.

New agents

None of the wide range of biological agents under development (Chapter 3) has yet been studied in children.

Given the likely central role of gut bacteria in its pathogenesis, research is being targeted at alteration of the intestinal flora in the management of Crohn's disease. In one small preliminary open label study, *Lactobacillus GG* appeared to improve the outcome of mild-to moderate Crohn's disease in children.[512] Further studies are underway.

Surgery

A study of 522 patients with Crohn's disease, diagnosed at less than 21 years of age and followed up for a mean of 7 years, revealed that 70% required surgery.[513] Indications include medically resistant disease, strictures, abscesses, fistulae and perianal disease. Surgery is generally most effective in those with localized disease.[514] However, in a retrospective study of 30 children, 50% had recurrent disease by two years after surgery.[515] Well-timed surgery can allow better symptom control, growth and progress through puberty.[516,517]

Oro-facial granulomatosis

Treatment of the swollen lips and ulceration of orofacial granulomatosis is notoriously difficult (Chapter 6). Enteral nutrition has been found to be effective in a case report.[518] Other approaches include a cinammon-free and benzoate-free diet, topical steroid or 5-ASA preparations, antibiotics, systemic steroids and immunosuppressants, but none, unsurprisingly, has been the subject of controlled evaluation.

Future developments

As will be clear from this chapter, there are few good quality data to supply the evidence base for treating this difficult disease in children. Thus, as in many diseases in children, therapeutic practice is largely based on extrapolation from studies in adults. It remains to be seen how the increasing number of novel treatments under development will impact on children.

Drug licensing authorities are now giving both financial ('carrot') and legal ('stick') incentives to companies to include children in studies of novel drugs.[519] Since December 2000, the FDA have required all companies to include paediatric data in all new drug applications as well as applications to extend the indications for use of existing treatments. In a separate act, the FDA has permitted companies to extend their period of exclusive marketing rights by six months if they include data obtained in paediatric studies. While there are guidelines in Europe, these are not enforceable by law and there is no financial incentive to abide by them (European Agency for the Evaluation of Medicinal Products, ICH Topic E11, 1999).

Conclusions

While the principles of treatment of Crohn's disease in children are generally similar to those in adults with the disease (Figure 8.1), special attention must be paid to the complications specific to children, particularly poor growth and delayed puberty. Although the use of enteral nutrition appears to be an effective way of minimizing these complications, longer-term studies are required to confirm this benefit. The major challenge over the next few years will to find the best treatments to prevent relapse once remission with enteral feeds or steroids has been achieved and to allow optimal health, growth and development.

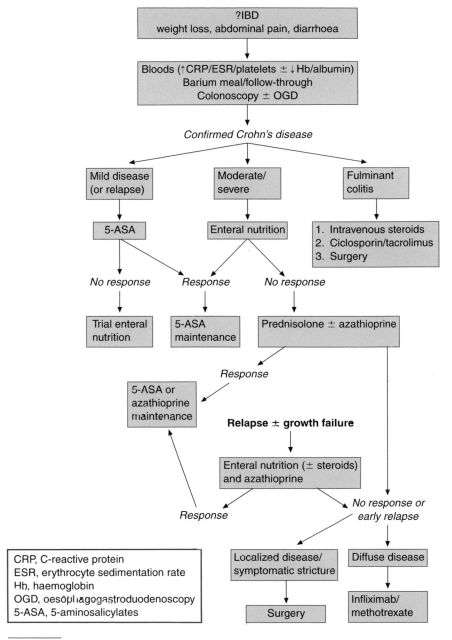

Figure 8.1 *Management of suspected Crohn's disease in childhood.*

chapter 9

Management of complications and manifestations of Crohn's disease

Introduction

Crohn's disease is associated with a variety of intestinal and extraintestinal manifestations which result from its systemic nature. These can be distinguished from complications resulting directly from the pathophysiology of the gut disease or from its treatment (Table 9.1).

Intestinal complications

Undernutrition

Prevalence and causes
As shown in Table 9.2, nutritional deficiency is common in Crohn's; its causes are multi-factorial and summarized in Table 9.3.[520]

Poor oral intake can arise from abdominal pain, nausea, vomiting or diarrhoea;[369] indeed, many patients feel that by excluding certain dietary constituents, which may, like dairy products, be of high nutritional value, they can reduce their symptoms.[27] Inflammation and/or surgery can result in malabsorption due to loss of mucosal surface area. More specifically, terminal ileal disease or resection can lead to a failure to absorb B_{12} and bile salts; severe bile salt deficiency itself can cause fat malabsorption. Active mucosal inflammation may provoke loss of fluid, blood, protein and minerals; it also increases metabolic turnover and can lead to folate deficiency. Finally, drug-related nutrient deficiencies may occur. These include folate deficiency in patients on

Table 9.1 Intestinal and extraintestinal manifestations and complications of Crohn's disease.

System	Resulting problem	Manifestation of disease	Complication of disease or its treatment
Intestinal	Undernutrition		*
	Short bowel syndrome		*
	Carcinoma		*
Joints/bones	Inflammatory arthropathy	*	
	Sacroiliitis	*	
	Ankylosing spondylitis	*	
	Clubbing	*	
	Osteoporosis		*
Eyes	Episcleritis and scleritis	*	
	Uveitis	*	
Skin	Erythema nodosum	*	
	Pyoderma gangrenosum	*	
Mouth		*	
Liver	Fatty change		*
	Chronic active hepatitis	*	
	Granulomatous hepatitis	*	
	Cirrhosis	*	
	Amyloid		*
Biliary tract	Cholesterol gallstones (terminal ileal Crohn's disease or resection)		*
	Sclerosing cholangitis	*	
	Cholangiocarcinoma	*	
Kidneys	Uric acid stones (total colitis/ileostomy)		*
	Oxalate stones (terminal ileal Crohn's disease or resection)		*
	Amyloid		*
Blood	Anaemia (iron, B12, folate deficiency)		*
	Arterial and venous thrombosis		*
Constitutional	Weight loss		*
	Growth retardation (children)		*
Psychosocial			*

Table 9.2 Prevalence of nutritional deficiencies in Crohn's disease.[520]

	Inpatient (%)	Outpatient (%)
Weight loss	65–75	54
Hypoalbuminaemia	25–80	0
Anaemia	60–80	54
Iron	25–50	37–53
Folic acid	54–62	10
Vitamin B_{12}	48	3–4
Calcium	13	ND
Magnesium	14–33	ND
Vitamin A	11–50	ND
Vitamin D	23–75	NR
Vitamin E	0	ND
Vitamin K	NR	ND
Zinc	40	1
Copper	ND	1–3
Selenium	NR	NR

ND, not determined.
NR, described but prevalence not recorded.

Table 9.3 Causes of undernutrition in Crohn's disease.[369]

Poor oral intake	Restricted diet due to pain, nausea, diarrhoea Disease-induced
Malabsorption	Decreased absorptive area (disease or surgery) Bacterial overgrowth Bile salt deficiency Drug-induced
Increased intestinal and nutrient loss	Protein-losing enteropathy Electrolyte, mineral and trace element loss Blood loss
Increased utilization and requirements	Inflammation Infection Increased intestinal cell turnover
Drugs	Corticosteroids Sulphasalazine, methotrexate, cholestyramine, colestipol (folate deficiency)

long-term sulphasalazine or methotrexate, and depletion of vitamin K as well as folate by ion-exchange resins such as cholestyramine (Chapter 3).

Monitoring of undernutrition (Table 9.4)

Weight should be measured regularly and used with height to calculate the BMI (weight (kg)/height (m)^2) (Chapter 6). In sick patients and those with

Table 9.4 Establishing and assessing undernutrition.

Clinical assessment	History	Anorexia Dietary history including assessment of calorie and nitrogen intake (dietitian) Food and fluid chart
	Examination	Muscle wasting Oedema Vitamin and mineral deficiencies such as angular stomatitis (iron)
	Height (m) and weight (kg)	BMI (weight/height^2) (<19) or a loss of >10% weight in 3 months

	Skin thickness (useful if patient oedematous or unable to be weighed)	Mid-upper arm circumference
		  men: <30 cm
		  women: <26 cm
		Mid-triceps skin-fold thickness
		  men: <8 mm
		  women: <17 mm

Objective measurements	Blood tests	Haemoglobin Albumin Folate, B$_{12}$, ferritin Calcium, magnesium, zinc Essential fatty acids Fat-soluble vitamins (A, D, E, K)
	Basal metabolic rate (BMR)	BMR: Harris–Benedict calculation[523] (see text) with adjustments as the clinical situation demands
	Nitrogen requirement	Nitrogen requirements: Elia[524] (see text) with adjustments as the clinical situation demands
Functional assessment	Muscle power	Grip strength

oedema, mid-upper arm circumference, triceps skin-fold thickness[521] and functional measures such as grip strength[522] should be monitored. Abnormalities of blood count and low serum albumin can be related to active Crohn's and sepsis, and often correlate poorly with undernutrition. Haematinics (B_{12}, folate and ferritin), minerals (calcium, magnesium and zinc), essential fatty acids and fat-soluble vitamins (A, D, E, and K) should be checked regularly in patients with extensive small bowel disease or resection (Table 9.4). Calculations of nitrogen balance and basal metabolic rate (for example, Harris–Benedict calculation) are desirable in patients needing enteral or parenteral nutritional supplementation.[523,524]

Management

The options available for nutritional support for undernourished patients with Crohn's disease range from supplemental sip feeding to parenteral nutrition (Chapter 5).

Enteral nutrition. Whenever possible, the oral route should be used for feeding since it is safer (Table 9.5) and maintains gut mucosal function better

Table 9.5 Complications of enteral and intravenous feeding.[369]

	Enteral feeding	*Parenteral feeding*
Placement of feeding catheters	Dislodgement or incorrect placement of nasogastric, PEG and PEJ tubes, infections at skin sites, aspiration pneumonia	Pneumothorax, subclavian or carotid artery puncture, haemothorax, subclavian vein thrombosis, thoracic duct injury, tunnelled-line related infection, septicaemia
Metabolic complications	Refeeding syndrome: hypokalaemia, hyponatraemia hypophosphataemia, hypomagnesaemia	Fluid overload, refeeding syndrome, hyperglycaemia, hyperosmolarity, liver function test derangement, metabolic bone disease, hypercalcaemia, renal stones
GI side-effects	Vomiting, diarrhoea, abdominal cramps	Biliary sludge, acalculous cholecystitis, pancreatitis

PEG, percutaneous endoscopic gastrostomy; PEJ, percutaneous endoscopic jejunostomy.

than parenteral nutrition.[369] If oral supplementation is poorly tolerated, nasogastric or PEG (percutaneous endoscopic gastrostomy) feeding can be used; the latter is safe in Crohn's.[525] Only if insufficient nutrients would be absorbed from the gut to meet demands, for example if vomiting, subacute obstruction, ileus or short bowel syndrome are present, should intravenous nutrition be considered. Regular monitoring (Table 9.4) is necessary to avoid complications of enteral feeding (Table 9.5) and to ensure that it is effective. Polymeric diets are preferred except in patients with extensive resections or inflammation, when a monomeric diet may be better absorbed (Table 5.1).[526]

Parenteral nutrition (TPN). Intravenous nutrition may be required in the short term perioperatively to maintain nutrition and to enhance wound healing,[371] and in the longer term for patients with short bowel syndrome (see below). Longer-term TPN is usually given by a tunnelled central venous catheter, while for periods of less than 10 days, a peripherally placed venous catheter or non-tunnelled line can be used; scrupulous asepsis is essential. Complications are shown in Table 9.5.

Home parenteral nutrition, sometimes for many years, may be needed in well-motivated and individually trained patients with short bowel syndrome.[369] The quality of life of patients on long-term TPN is frequently reduced to a level comparable with patients receiving dialysis for chronic renal failure: many patients become socially isolated and depressed.[527]

Refeeding syndrome. One of the complications of starting either enteral or parenteral feeding in very malnourished patients is the refeeding syndrome.[528,529] This comprises severe hypophosphataemia, hypomagnesaemia, hypokalaemia, abnormal glucose metabolism and thiamine deficiency in the first few days of feeding, and is potentially lethal (Table 9.5).[528] It can be averted by instituting feeding slowly and careful monitoring of phosphate, magnesium, potassium and glucose.[528]

Short bowel syndrome

Definition, types and causes

The short bowel syndrome occurs when there is insufficient length of functioning intestine to allow adequate absorption of water, electrolytes and nutrients to maintain homeostasis.[530,531] If less than 200 cm of small bowel remain, undernutrition and/or fluid and electrolyte depletion will occur without appropriate treatment. The consequences of the short bowel

(a)   (b)

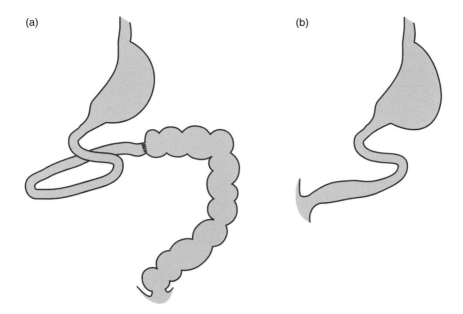

Figure 9.1 *Types of short bowel which may occur post-resection. (a) Jejunocolic anastomosis and (b) jejunostomy.*

syndrome depend upon the type and length of remaining small bowel and the presence or absence of a functioning colon.

The two commonest anatomical arrangements causing the short bowel syndrome are a jejunocolic anastomosis (jejunum–colon) and an end jejunostomy, in which some jejunum, the ileum and the colon have been removed (Figure 9.1). Crohn's disease accounts for at least half of patients with short bowel syndrome, other causes including superior mesenteric artery thrombosis and irradiation damage.

Physiological consequences and presentation (Table 9.6)

Salt and water balance. Jejunum–colon: Conservation of a normally functioning colon is advantageous as this organ absorbs sodium and water, magnesium, calcium[530] and short chain fatty acids derived from anaerobic bacterial fermentation; the latter make a small but important contribution to the patient's calorie supply.[531,532] For these reasons, patients with a preserved colon often appear well soon after their resection except for diarrhoea and/or steatorrhoea, but thereafter gradually become undernourished if untreated.

Table 9.6 Main clinical problems associated with short bowel syndrome.[530]

Problem	Jejunum–colon	Jejunostomy
Presentation	Gradual onset of diarrhoea and undernutrition	Immediate fluid depletion
Salt, water and magnesium deficiency	Uncommon long term	Common
Nutrient deficiencies	Common	Common
Oxalate renal stones	Common	None
Gall stones	Common	Common
Social problems	Offensive diarrhoea	Effluent leakage, skin excoriation and treatment dependence

Jejunostomy: Patients with a jejunostomy suffer immediately from large stomal losses of salt and water. Jejunostomy patients can be classified as net 'absorbers' or net 'secretors'.[530] Net absorbers absorb more water and sodium from their gut than they take orally, the excess absorption being from salivary, gastric and pancreaticobiliary secretions. These patients have a stomal output of about 2 litres/day. They usually have more than 100 cm of residual jejunum and can be managed with oral sodium and water supplements. Net secretors, in contrast, have a shorter length of residual jejunum and lose more salt and water from their stoma than they take by mouth. The stomal output of secretors may be 4 to 8 litres/day, with the output being highest after food and drink.[533] These patients usually require parenteral salt and water replacement.

Other physiological consequences of short bowel syndrome

Gastrointestinal secretions. Extensive small bowel resection causes hypergastrinaemia, possibly as a result of reduced intestinal catabolism of gastrin.[534] Consequent gastric acid hypersecretion can cause peptic ulceration, reduced fat absorption as a result of bile salt precipitation[535] and reduced pancreatic enzyme function.

Gastrointestinal motility. Gastric emptying and small bowel transit are rapid in patients with a jejunostomy and normal in those with a retained colon, probably as a result of changes in plasma concentrations of peptide YY, a product of L cells in the colon.[536]

Absorptive function. If more than 60 cm of terminal ileum is resected, vitamin B_{12} deficiency may occur.[537] If more than 100 cm of terminal ileum is removed, bile salt malabsorption cannot be matched by increased hepatic synthesis of bile salts so that fat malabsorption results.[311] Bile salt malabsorption also leads to a risk of gall stones and enteric hyperoxaluria (see below).

Intestinal adaptation. After intestinal resection, adaptation may gradually improve absorption of water, electrolytes and nutrients.[538] Mechanisms include gut hormone-mediated increases in absorptive area (structural adaptation) and gastrointestinal transit time (functional adaptation).[530]

Investigation

Assessment of residual small intestine. The remaining small bowel length should be measured, if possible, at surgery without overstretching the bowel. Alternatively, an attempt can be made to assess small bowel length on barium follow-through examination.[539]

Fluid and electrolyte balance. Daily body weight and accurate fluid balance, including stomal output in jejunostomy patients, are essential. Initially, serum potassium, magnesium and creatinine, together with urinary sodium concentration, should be measured daily, later twice a week and then less often if the patient requires long-term intravenous fluids. Patients with a high stomal output are at risk of hypotension, prerenal failure and magnesium depletion with consequent fatigue, depression, ataxia, cardiac arrhythmias, tetany and convulsions.

Nutritional status. A body mass index (BMI) <19, unintentional weight loss >10% or a mid-arm circumference of less than 26 cm for a woman or 30 cm for a man[540] each indicate undernourishment (Table 9.4).

Management of specific clinical problems (Table 9.7)

Salt and water depletion.
Jejunum–colon: In view of its large absorptive capacity, patients with the colon preserved rarely need salt or water supplements. However, if patients do become sodium depleted, a glucose-saline drink is usually sufficient.

Jejunostomy: For patients with a high output jejunostomy, sodium and water depletion are prevented and treated initially with intravenous normal saline. The patient is kept nil by mouth since feeding increases stomal output as a result of increased endogenous secretions. Over a few days, intravenous fluids are tapered while food and hypotonic drinks are restricted. Patients with stomal losses <1.2 litres/day can usually maintain salt and water balance by adding extra salt to the diet and limiting oral fluid intake to 1 litre/day. Patients with higher stomal losses need a glucose-saline solution containing sodium at 90–100 mmol/l to match its concentration in jejunostomy effluent. In hot weather, additional salt is necessary.

Other measures for short bowel syndrome

Antidiarrhoeal drugs. Loperamide and codeine phosphate, by reducing intestinal motility and increasing salt absorption, can reduce stoma output by 30%.[541] In patients with short bowel syndrome and rapid small bowel transit, high doses of loperamide (for example 24 mg/day) may be needed. The drug should be given before food, as intestinal output rises substantially after meals.[530]

Cholestyramine. This is used in patients with intact colons to combat bile salt-induced diarrhoea (Chapter 3), but can, in patients with extensive ileal disease or resection, induce steatorrhoea by worsening bile-salt depletion.[311]

Inhibition of gastric acid secretion. H_2 receptor antagonists and proton pump inhibitors help reduce jejunostomy output.[542]

Somatostatin/octreotide. Both these agents reduce salivary, gastric and pancreaticobiliary secretions and delay gut transit. Since somatostatin needs to be given by continuous infusion,[543] octreotide subcutaneously twice or three times daily before food is the preferred agent in patients with salt and water loss which persists despite the above measures.[544]

Table 9.7 Principles of treatment of short bowel syndrome.

Problem	Jejunum–colon	Jejunostomy
Salt and water deficiency	Usually unnecessary	Intravenous saline, restrict oral fluid, glucose-saline drinks, loperamide, PPI, octreotide
Magnesium deficiency	Usually unnecessary	Salt and water repletion, magnesium oxide, 1-alpha calcidol
Vitamin deficiencies	B_{12}, thiamine, A, D, E, K	B_{12}, thiamine, A, D, E, K
Other deficiencies	Usually unnecessary	Selenium, zinc, sunflower oil topically
Protein energy malnutrition	High carbohydrate/low fat diet, sip-feeds, enteral feeding, medium chain triglycerides, sunflower oil topically	Sip-feeds, enteral feeding, high fat diet if possible, TPN if necessary
Diarrhoea	Limit food intake, loperamide, cholestyramine, PPI	See salt and water deficiency as above
Hyperoxaluria	Low oxalate/high calcium/low fat diet, medium chain triglycerides, possibly cholestyramine	Unnecessary

PPI, proton pump inhibitors; TPN, total parenteral nutrition.

Magnesium deficiency. Hypomagnesaemia occurs as a result of loss of its main absorptive sites (distal small bowel and colon),[545] increased renal magnesium excretion as a result of salt depletion-induced secondary hyperaldosteronism[546] and reduced secretion and function of parathyroid hormone (PTH).[547]

Treatment starts with restoration of salt and water. The most widely used magnesium preparation is magnesium oxide, preferably being given at night when intestinal transit is slowest.[530] In patients not responding, oral

1-α hydroxycholecalciferol is usually effective.[548] Intravenous magnesium is necessary in symptomatic patients.

Other vitamin and mineral deficiencies. Patients with more than 60 cm of terminal ileum removed need long-term hydroxocobalamin injections. It may be necessary to counteract reduced absorption of fat-soluble vitamins (A, D, E and K) by appropriate parenteral replacement therapy. Essential fatty acid deficiency can be prevented by rubbing sunflower oil into the skin.[549]

Selenium replacement is needed in patients with a jejunostomy and/or on long-term parenteral nutrition.[550] Zinc deficiency should be sought and treated intravenously or orally in patients with large stool volume.[551]

Protein-energy malnutrition. Because of malabsorption, patients who can be maintained on an oral diet need a higher energy intake than normal subjects: this is given as oral sip-feeds or enteral feeding at night through a nasogastric or percutaneous endoscopic gastrostomy tube.[525] If these measures fail, parenteral nutrition is necessary. The management of patients requiring long-term home parenteral administration is beyond the scope of this book.[552]

Jejunum–colon: As unabsorbed long chain fatty acids reduce transit time and fluid absorption in the colon[553] and cause excessive oxalate absorption there (see below), a low fat diet is theoretically best for patients with small bowel resection. However, a low fat diet is unpalatable, reduces energy supply and increases the risk of calcium, magnesium and essential fatty acid deficiency.[554] In patients in whom energy intake cannot be maintained with plentiful carbohydrates, medium chain triglycerides may be needed.[554]

Jejunostomy: Because patients with a jejunostomy absorb a constant proportion of dietary nitrogen, energy and fat, increased fat in the diet increases energy provision, provides essential fatty acids and improves palatability.[556]

Prevention of drug malabsorption. Patients with a short bowel syndrome may need higher doses of drugs such as thyroxine, warfarin[557] and digoxin.[558]

Small bowel transplantation. Small bowel transplantation is neither sufficiently developed nor widely available to be routinely applicable in the tiny minority of patients with short bowel syndrome due to Crohn's refractory to all other therapies; furthermore, it is accompanied by a risk of recurrence in the transplanted bowel.[559]

Social problems. All patients with short bowel syndrome have diarrhoea and/or steatorrhoea. The effluent from a jejunostomy is not offensive, but frequent bag changing may be necessary and leakage of the fluid can cause local skin soreness. Despite these problems, most patients with a short bowel have a normal BMI in the long term, work full time and look after their families unaided.

Carcinoma of the colon and rectum

Incidence and risk factors
Patients with ulcerative colitis (UC) have an increased risk of colorectal carcinoma (CRC). [560]

The risk of CRC in Crohn's disease has not been as well defined but is probably about 7% over 20 years, a figure resembling that for UC.[561,562] Risk factors other than duration of Crohn's include older age, male sex, right-sided colonic or ileocolonic disease, a family history of CRC and co-existent sclerosing cholangitis.[81,563–565] Carcinomas tend to arise in areas affected by Crohn's, particularly when these are bypassed (Chapter 4).[566] Most patients with Crohn's-related CRC have dysplasia in adjacent (86%) or more distant mucosa (41%), supporting a dysplasia-carcinoma sequence as for UC.[566]

Prevention
Cancer prevention in Crohn's disease includes two main strategies, neither yet evidence-based.[560]

The first is to prevent malignant transformation, for example by using 5-ASA drugs and/or folic acid, as in UC,[567,568] or by resecting chronically inflamed segments of colon and avoiding creating bypasses when operating (Chapter 4).[72]

The second approach involves colonoscopic screening to detect dysplasia or cancer at an early stage. In the largest screening programme reported to date, 16% of 259 patients with Crohn's colitis had dysplasia or carcinoma during a 20-year follow-up.[81] This protocol involved taking four biopsies every 10 cm as well as from all strictures and polypoidal masses at least 2-yearly, and more frequently in patients with alarm symptoms or previous dysplasia.[81]

Colonoscopic screening programmes have not yet been shown to reduce mortality from CRC in UC and there is not yet evidence on which to base screening recommendations in Crohn's colitis. Some of the problems associated with colonoscopic screening in Crohn's disease resemble those for UC, for example the discomfort, hazards and expense of the procedure, and the difficulty of defining the grade of dysplasia and its natural history.[560] In addition, full colonoscopy in Crohn's colitis may be impossible if strictures are present[81] and the end product of colectomy in Crohn's disease, a permanent ileostomy, may be harder for patients to accept than an ileoanal pouch, the usual result of surgery in UC.

Small intestinal carcinoma

Small bowel cancers are extremely rare in patients without Crohn's disease. The magnitude of the risk in patients with Crohn's is difficult to evaluate as a large enough study has not been performed.[564] In one study of 600 patients with Crohn's disease, four small bowel cancers were diagnosed over 16 years, giving an apparent relative risk of 86-fold compared with the general population.[569] In Crohn's disease, most small bowel cancers occur in the diseased ileum;[569,570] they have also been reported in fistulae, bypassed bowel and strictureplasty sites.[569,571–573] Small bowel cancers usually present with obstruction and are treated surgically.

Anal carcinoma

Although this squamous cell lesion is thought to arise in chronically damaged mucosa, its incidence even in Crohn's disease is low: in an 18-year study of nearly 10 000 patients with IBD, only two cases occurred.[574] Nevertheless, malignancy should be considered in any non-healing perineal sinus or fistula, with biopsy and subsequent wide excision of the tract, chemotherapy and radiotherapy as appropriate.[575]

Extraintestinal manifestations of Crohn's disease

Extra-intestinal manifestations of Crohn's disease occur more often in patients with colonic or ileocolonic than small intestinal disease.[576] They most frequently affect the skin, joints and eyes, with the presence of one manifestation significantly increasing the probability of others.[576] Bacterial antigens, immune complexes and cryoproteins are postulated as pathogenic factors.[577] Similar extraintestinal manifestations may occur with ulcerative colitis, enteric infections or non-intestinal inflammatory diseases.[577] Since several of the extraintestinal manifestations of Crohn's flare in parallel with its activity in the gut,[578] treatment involves not only therapy of the manifestation itself, but also measures to reduce intestinal inflammation.

Joint disease

Joint disease occurs in 10–30% of patients with IBD, the prevalence increasing with disease duration.[576] Peripheral arthritis mirrors the activity of Crohn's disease, but ankylosing spondylitis and sacroiliitis do not.[577]

Inflammatory arthropathy (peripheral arthritis)

Presentation. In this condition the large peripheral joints show asymmetrical swelling without joint destruction or bony erosion. Type 1 'pauciarticular' disease involves fewer than five joints, and type 2 'polyarticular' disease five joints or more.[579] Type 1 disease is more commonly associated (76%) with active IBD than type 2 (42%).[579] The type of arthritis is determined by HLA genotype.[580]

Management. Treatment of the underlying gut inflammation often leads to remission of joint symptoms. NSAIDs can relieve pain in the short term, but may exacerbate intestinal inflammation.[34] Whether selective COX2 inhibitors will be better tolerated than conventional NSAIDs by patients with Crohn's is not yet clear,[36] although a recent small series is reassuring.[581] Joint injection with corticosteroids may be helpful. Furthermore, by analogy with ankylosing spondylitis (see below) and rheumatoid arthritis, it is often suggested that sulphasalazine (rather than other 5-ASA drugs) may ameliorate joint disease.[582] Finally, since patients with an intact ileocaecal region have an increased incidence of arthritis compared with those who have undergone ileocaecal resection, there may conceivably be a case for right hemicolectomy in such patients whose arthropathy is refractory to medical treatment.[583]

Ankylosing spondylitis and sacroiliitis

Presentation. These conditions affect about 3% of patients with Crohn's[576] and are unrelated to intestinal inflammation. They may present years before the onset of gut symptoms. Unlike ankylosing spondylitis in the general population, only 35% of patients with Crohn's are HLA-B27 positive, and the male to female ratio is approximately equal.[576]

Management. Physiotherapy and NSAIDs increase mobility. Sulphasalazine (but not other 5-ASA drugs) may ameliorate joint as well as bowel disease: its sulphapyridine component is postulated to have immunomodulatory as well as antibiotic effects.[584] Recent data indicate that infliximab is extremely effective in ameliorating the symptoms of patients with severe ankylosing spondylitis.[695]

Clubbing of nails

Clubbing occurs more frequently in active than inactive Crohn's, the incidence being 15–60%. The pathogenesis is unknown and clubbing may regress with resection, only to recur if the gut disease relapses.[585]

Eyes

While uveitis occurs more frequently in UC, scleritis and episcleritis are more common in Crohn's.[586] In one study, ocular disease was found more frequently in patients with ileocolonic or colonic disease (24%) than in those with isolated small bowel Crohn's (3%).[587] Furthermore, ocular symptoms were more common in patients with arthritis or arthralgia (30%) than in those without (7%).[587,588] As with joint disease (see above), ocular inflammation appears to be strongly HLA-associated.[588]

Episcleritis and scleritis

Presentation. In episcleritis, inflammation below the conjunctiva may cause an inflammatory nodule (Figure 9.2). Symptoms include burning, itching and tenderness over the nodule. Ocular examination shows locally dilated blood vessels and a nodule. Scleritis is more serious and fortunately rarer, causing perforation in severe cases.

Treatment. Both conditions require prompt specialist ophthalmological treatment; this includes corticosteroid eye drops. Active intestinal Crohn's also needs appropriate therapy (Chapters 3 and 6).

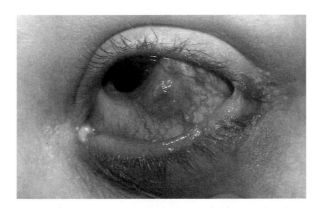

Figure 9.2 *Episcleritis.*

Anterior uveitis

Presentation. Acute inflammation of the anterior chamber of the eye causes severe ocular pain, photophobia, blurring of vision, lacrimation, headache and circumcorneal redness. The pupil is initially small from spasm of the iris and later becomes irregular as a result of adhesions (synechiae) within the anterior chamber; these may prevent drainage of aqueous fluid and cause glaucoma. Rarely, uveitis is asymptomatic.[589] Slit lamp examination reveals pus in the anterior chamber (hypopyon) and white corneal precipitates.

Treatment. Prompt ophthalmological referral is essential. Treatment consists of corticosteroid drops to reduce inflammation, with cyclopentolate drops to dilate the pupil and reduce the likelihood of adhesions. Analgesia and treatment of active intestinal disease (Chapters 3 and 6) are also needed.

Skin

The incidence of erythema nodosum is about 8% and of pyoderma gangrenosum 1% in patients with Crohn's disease.[576] Both conditions may precede a diagnosis of Crohn's. In those patients with treatment-resistant erythema nodosum and in all with pyoderma gangrenosum, dermatological referral is advisable.

Erythema nodosum

Presentation. Erythema nodosum is characterized by the appearance over a few days of tender, bluish-red nodules with diameter up to 5 cm; their

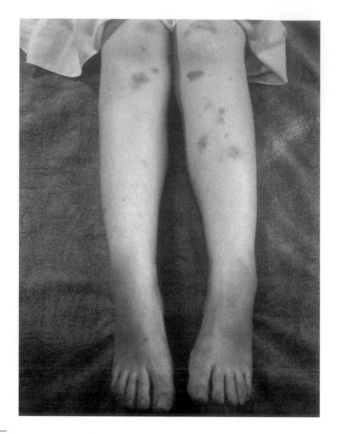

Figure 9.3 *Erythema nodosum.*

commonest site is the anterior shin (Figure 9.3). The lesions usually coincide with a flare-up of disease activity, fading when remission occurs. Erythema nodosum is more common in women than men, and in patients with ileocolonic and colonic disease.[578] Biopsy, although rarely necessary, reveals a panniculitis or non-specific vasculitis.

Management. Hydrocortisone cream (1%) may give local relief, but more important is active management of the intestinal disease (Chapters 3 and 6).

Pyoderma gangrenosum

Presentation. Pyoderma gangrenosum begins as a small pustule which expands to cause deep, discrete ulcerated areas with necrotic bluish margins (Figure 9.4). Lesions may be multiple and often occur at operation scars and

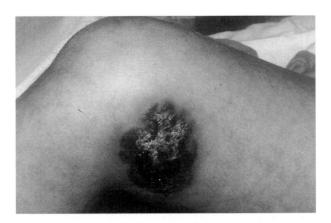

Figure 9.4 *Pyoderma gangrenosum.*

sites of trauma; they are most commonly located on the lower legs. Pyoderma does not mirror relapses of intestinal disease. Biopsy is not routinely necessary, but shows inflammation with a perivascular leukocyte infiltrate; special staining shows the presence of immunoglobulin and complement components.

Management. Intralesional, oral and intravenous corticosteroids, aminosalicylates, immunosuppression and dapsone have all been tried with variable results.[590] Some patients respond, anecdotally, to ciclosporin,[591] intravenous heparin[592] and infliximab.[593] Colectomy improves refractory pyoderma in about one-third of patients with UC and may be a last resort in patients with Crohn's colitis and treatment-resistant pyoderma.[590]

Mouth

Aphthous ulceration

Aphthous ulceration is no commoner in patients with Crohn's than in the general population, occurring in 5–15% of people.[577] However, in Crohn's disease the ulcers are often larger, deeper and less painful than in the normal population and may parallel disease activity.[577] They need to be distinguished from oral Crohn's disease (Chapters 2 and 6).

Hepatobiliary disease

Transiently abnormal liver function tests (LFT) are common in active IBD, partly as a result of malnutrition and sepsis. The prevalence of chronic liver disease is approximately 5% in both Crohn's disease and UC, the commonest being primary sclerosing cholangitis. When liver disease occurs in Crohn's, it is usually in patients with extensive colonic involvement.[594,595] To expedite diagnosis, liver function tests should be checked at least annually in all IBD patients.

Primary sclerosing cholangitis

Presentation. Primary sclerosing cholangitis (PSC) is a chronic cholestatic disease resulting from inflammatory and obliterative stricturing of the intra- and/or extrahepatic biliary tree.[595,596] The initial stages are asymptomatic, patients often being diagnosed from minor abnormalities in LFTs. Symptomatic patients present with fatigue, jaundice, pruritus, right upper quadrant pain and weight loss.[596] Progression occurs over 5–15 years and leads to cholestasis, ascending cholangitis, cholangiocarcinoma and cirrhosis with resulting portal hypertension and liver failure.[577]

In a study of patients with Crohn's, 10 out of 262 (4%) had abnormal LFTs; one patient had non-specific reactive hepatitis and the other nine PSC.[594] Of the latter, three patients had large duct PSC, five had small duct PSC (normal cholangiogram, the diagnosis made on liver biopsy) and one was unclassified. The mean age at diagnosis was 35 years, seven were female and two male. All nine patients had colonic disease and two developed colorectal carcinoma.[594]

Investigation. The most common LFT abnormalities are raised alkaline phosphatase and bilirubin. Later changes include a fall in serum albumin and clotting abnormalities.[596] Some patients have low level titres of antinuclear and smooth muscle antibodies; pANCA (Chapter 1) is positive in 60–80% of patients with PSC complicating UC, but figures relating to Crohn's disease are unavailable.[597]

Endoscopic retrograde cholangio-pancreatography (ERCP) shows multiple strictures with focal dilatation of intra- and extrahepatic ducts in large-duct disease (Figure 9.5).[596] Pancreaticobiliary MRI is progressively replacing ERCP for diagnosis as it is non-invasive and risk-free.[598] Liver biopsy is unnecessary in patients with clear-cut large duct PSC, but in small duct disease shows bile ducts narrowed by dense concentric fibrosis of their submucosa and outer layer giving the classical appearance of 'onion skin' fibrosis.[595]

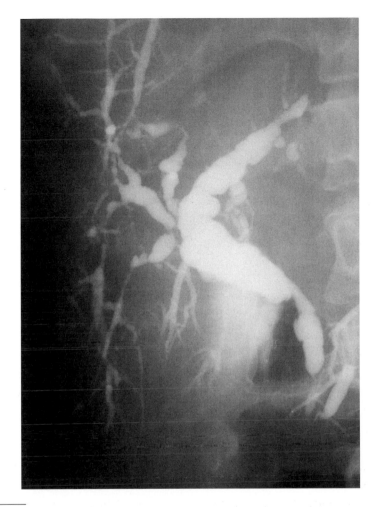

Figure 9.5 *Endoscopic retrograde cholangio-pancreatography appearances of primary sclerosing cholangitis.*

Management. Ursodeoxycholic acid (10–15 mg/kg per day) improves pruritus and jaundice.[599] Higher doses (up to 20–25 mg/kg per day) may delay progression of PSC as judged by liver biopsy.[600]

In patients with acute cholangitis complicating PSC, antibiotics such as ciprofloxacin are used, but there is no evidence to support long-term prophylactic antibiotics. Similarly, immunosuppressive treatment has not been shown to be of benefit. Dominant large duct strictures can be stented at ERCP or percutanous transhepatic cholangiography.

However, the only treatment which clearly improves prognosis is ortho-topic liver transplantation (OLT). The indications for OLT are progressive jaundice, refractory pruritus, biliary dysplasia and the absence of cholangio-carcinoma.[595] Four-year survival after OLT is 70%.[595] Some patients undergo-ing OLT experience a remission of their IBD, probably as a result of the necessary immunosuppressive treatment.[601]

Whether or not OLT has been performed, PSC increases the risk of colo-rectal carcinoma in Crohn's disease and screening by yearly colonoscopy and multiple biopsies is recommended.[594] Furthermore, a recent report sug-gests that oral ursodeoxycholic acid may provide some protection against this complication.[602]

Cholangiocarcinoma

Cholangiocarcinoma complicating PSC in Crohn's seems to be rare in com-parison with UC, in which there is an incidence of 0.5%: there are only two case reports.[603,604]

Patients present with progressive cholestatic jaundice and ERCP or MRI shows a biliary stricture, which may be difficult to differentiate from PSC. Bile and brush cytology can confirm malignancy, but each has low sensitivity.[605] In some patients, the diagnosis is made only on autopsy or from an explanted liver at OLT.[606] The prognosis is poor, with a median survival of only nine months.[595] Surgical excision is rarely feasible and OLT is contra-indicated because of rapid tumour recurrence in the graft.[607] Chemotherapy and radio-therapy are of little benefit and treatment is essentially palliative; stenting is used to relieve jaundice and antibiotics are given for acute cholangitis.[608]

Granulomatous hepatitis

Granulomas are often found in the liver biopsies of patients with Crohn's who have elevated serum alkaline phosphatase and γ-glutamyl-transferase, but they are of no clinical significance unless associated with PSC.[595]

Chronic active hepatitis

Chronic active hepatitis (CAH) has been associated with UC rather than Crohn's disease.[609] However, interface hepatitis or piecemeal necrosis is some-times found on liver biopsy in patients with the bile duct changes of PSC seen at ERCP or on MRI.[596] The implication is that the many presumed cases of CAH may in fact be PSC; CAH should not be diagnosed except in the pres-ence of normal cholangiography and appropriate serological abnormalities.[595]

Extraintestinal complications of disease

These complications arise directly as a result of the disease itself or of its treatment.[577]

Hepatobiliary disease

Gall stones

Incidence and pathogenesis. Gall stones occur in up to 35% of patients with ileitis, ileal resection or intestinal bypass due to Crohn's.[610] In patients with ileal disease or resection, bile salt depletion as a result of their reduced ileal absorption leads to supersaturation of biliary cholesterol and the formation of gall stones. A further pathogenic factor may be impaired gallbladder contractility as a consequence of intestinal inflammation or resection.[611]

Management. The management of gall stones complicating Crohn's resembles that for patients without the disease. However, abdominal pain in patients with gall stones may be difficult to distinguish from that due to intestinal strictures. Furthermore, laparoscopic cholecystectomy may be hazardous in patients with adhesions due to previous surgery for Crohn's. Lastly, cholecystectomy carries an increased risk of causing bile salt-induced diarrhoea in patients with terminal ileal Crohn's disease or resection.[612]

Fatty liver

Hepatic steatosis occurs in about 4% of patients with Crohn's and in up to 40% of those who have undergone colectomy.[613] In Crohn's disease, fatty liver may reflect poor nutrition, although other causes such as alcohol and diabetes mellitus may co-exist. The deposition of fat is usually macrovesicular and can be diffuse, periportal or centrilobular.[595] Treating the underlying intestinal disease and malnutrition ameliorates fatty change, although the condition does not appear to progress to cirrhosis.[595]

Amyloidosis

Incidence and presentation

The prevalence of amyloidosis in Crohn's disease is about 1%; it is four times more common in colonic than small intestinal disease,[614] and is associated particularly with chronic active disease.[615] The diagnosis is made at a mean age of 40 years, approximately 15 years after the onset of Crohn's.[614]

Deposition of amyloid may occur in the kidneys, liver, spleen, heart and bowel wall.[577,614] The commonest presentation is with nephrotic syndrome and progressive renal insufficiency.

Management
Diagnosis is confirmed by biopsy of affected tissue. In vivo scintigraphy using radiolabelled ^{123}I serum amyloid P component may help monitor treatment.[615]

Colchicine (0.5–3 mg/day) retards or reverses early renal dysfunction.[615] Intensive and long-term suppression of disease activity, for example with azathioprine, is essential; plasmapheresis has met with some success.[577,615] The course of Crohn's disease in patients requiring renal transplantation is often good, perhaps because of ongoing immunosuppressive treatment.[615]

Renal complications
The incidence of renal stones is 6–10% in patients with Crohn's, the two main types being oxalate and urate.[616] Rarely, calcium-predominant stones occur in patients with hypercalciuria due to corticosteroid therapy.[577] Patients usually present with renal or ureteric colic. General principles of treatment resemble those of patients without Crohn's and include analgesia, hydration, urinary alkalinization, lithotripsy and stone extraction.

Calcium oxalate stone disease

Pathogenesis. Oxalate is excreted in the urine as an end product of metabolism. Urinary oxalate is normally derived principally from glyoxylate, ascorbic acid and dietary oxalate. The commonest cause of secondary hyperoxaluria is enteric hyperoxaluria, in which hyperabsorption of dietary oxalate occurs in the colon of patients with bowel disorders complicated by malabsorption of fat, bile salts or both (Figure 9.6).[617,618]

Treatment. Preventive therapy in patients with enteric hyperoxaluria is restricted to those with established nephrolithiasis or extensive ileal resections.

Reducing dietary oxalate intake by avoidance of oxalate-rich foods and drinks (e.g. spinach, beetroot, rhubarb, chocolate, tea, coffee, cola drinks) reduces urinary oxalate output. Fat restriction reduces hyperoxaluria in

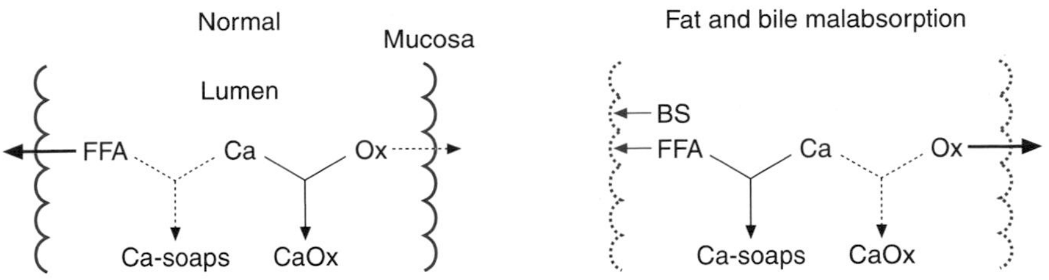

Figure 9.6 *Mechanism of enteric hyperoxaluria. In patients with steatorrhoea, non-absorbed fatty acids complex with calcium in the intestinal lumen allowing free oxalate to be absorbed from the colon; in addition, free fatty acids increase colonic mucosal permeability to oxalate. In patients with ileal Crohn's disease or ileal resection, bile salt malabsorption results in a bile salt-induced increase in colonic mucosal permeablity to oxalate. FFA, free fatty acids; Ca, calcium; Ox, oxalate; BS, bile salt.*

patients with steatorrhoea by decreasing luminal soap formation with calcium.[617]

Although calcium supplements, by precipitating oxalate in the gut lumen, reduce hyperoxaluria,[619] this may be counterbalanced by a rise in urinary calcium output so that the saturation product for urinary calcium oxalate is unchanged. Anion-exchange resins, such as cholestyramine (Chapter 3), bind oxalate, bile salts and fatty acids and reduce enteric hyperoxaluria.[619]

Urate stones

Urate stones occur as a result of fluid depletion, particularly in patients with high ileostomy output.[616] Treatment follows the general principles outlined above, with avoidance of fluid depletion and metabolic acidosis being important.[577]

Osteoporosis

Definition

Osteoporosis is characterized by a low bone mass, leading to enhanced bone fragility and risk of fracture.

The gold standard for measuring bone mineral density (BMD) is dual energy X-ray absorptiometry (DEXA) scanning. The number of standard deviations above or below the mean for an age-matched control is the Z score, while the T score is the number of standard deviations above or below the mean for young adults. It is important to distinguish between these two scores as older patients may fit the criteria for treatment with a T score of >-2.5 despite being within normal limits for their peer group.

Incidence and risk factors

Osteoporosis occurs in up to 40% of adults with Crohn's.[133,620] Although in one study the incidence of related 'fragility' fractures was 40% greater than in the general population,[621] in another it was not raised at all.[622] Reduced BMD is also common in children with IBD (Chapter 8).

Factors accounting for the high incidence of osteoporosis in Crohn's include intestinal inflammation, cumulative lifetime corticosteroid intake, low body mass index, inadequate intake and malabsorption of calcium and vitamin D, ileal resection, hypogonadism, smoking, reduced physical activity, gender and genetic variability.[577,620,623,624]

The effect of corticosteroids is cumulative and a lifetime prednisolene dose of 10 g yields a high risk of osteopenia.[625] A daily dose >7.5 mg prednisolone for greater than three months leads to significant bone loss, particularly in the early weeks of treatment.[625] BMD may be lower in men than women, firstly because women tend to be offered hormone replacement therapy (HRT) and secondly because Crohn's may affect testicular function and cause testosterone deficiency.[435] Genetic factors are likely to influence susceptibility to osteoporosis in IBD, one study indicating that allelic variability of the IL-1β gene increases the risk of this complication.[626]

Management (Figure 9.7)

Basic preventive advice for all patients with Crohn's disease includes avoiding smoking and excess alcohol, taking plenty of weight-bearing exercise and maintaining a body mass index of 20–25.[133] The daily calcium intake should be 1500 mg (a pint of skimmed milk contains 700 mg). If this level cannot be achieved, Calcichew tablets containing both calcium and vitamin D should be given, particularly if serum 25-hydroxy vitamin D levels are low.[133] Use of systemic corticosteroids should be restricted as far as possible. Topical formulations or controlled-release budesonide (Chapter 3) may be suitable alternatives. If avoidance of systemic steroid treatment is impossible, the addition of bisphosphonates and vitamin D may be necessary.[133]

BMD should be measured in middle-aged women either at the menopause or when first seen, in men at 55 years of age, at a lifetime cumulative dose of 10 g of prednisolone, and in all patients who have had fragility fractures.[133] If osteoporosis is found, as defined by a T score of >−2.5, or for those patients who have received corticosteroids, a T score of >−1.5,[133] active treatment should be started.

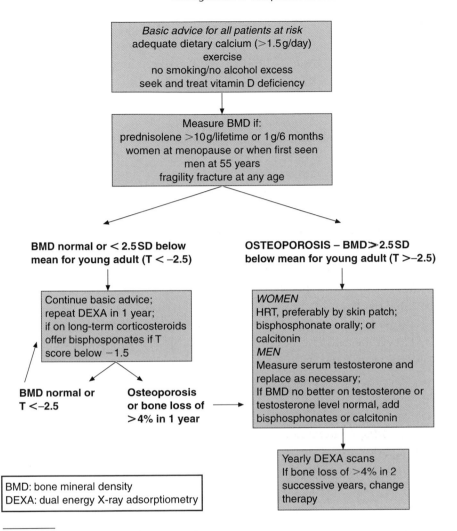

Figure 9.7 *Management of osteoporosis.*

For postmenopausal women, HRT should be given for at least 10 years, assuming patient compliance and the absence of contra-indications to its use. Special care with HRT is needed in patients with an intact uterus (because of the risk of inducing bleeding), migraine, stroke, myocardial infarction and thromboembolism.[627–629] Side-effects include nausea, bloating, abdominal cramps, breast enlargement and tenderness, depression, cholestatic jaundice and a 15–30% increase in the risk of breast cancer.[630,631]

For men with osteoporosis, testosterone levels should be measured[435] and corrected under specialist supervision if deficiency is found.[632]

If these measures do not improve DEXA scores, and in premenopausal women, treatment using bisphosphonates or calcitonin is advisable, particularly if fragility fractures have occurred.[632]

Bisphosphonates are given orally as etidronate (Didronel PMO with disodium etidronate (400 mg) with calcium carbonate (1.25 g) giving 14 days of both then 76 days of calcium only) or alendronate (Fosamax 10 mg daily or 70 mg/week). Side-effects include nausea, oesophageal inflammation, diarrhoea, constipation, abdominal pain, hypocalcaemia, hypophosphataemia, peripheral neuropathy, hypersensitivity reactions and blood dyscrasias. Contra-indications include renal impairment, pregnancy and breast-feeding, hypercalcaemia, hypercalciuria and conditions causing delayed oesophageal clearance. Patients should take 200 ml water with oral bisphosphonates, avoid food for two hours before or after taking the medication and remain upright for at least 30 minutes afterwards to ensure its rapid transit out of the oesophagus.

Intravenous disodium pamidronate is an alternative for patients intolerant of oral bisphosphonates. One effective dosage regime is 30 mg, infused over two hours, every three months[633] and another 15 mg/day (over two hours) for five days with courses repeated every three months as necessary.[634]

Calcitonin (100 units/day) can be given subcutaneously or intramuscularly with oral vitamin D and calcium as needed.[635] Side-effects include nausea, vomiting, parasthesiae, inflammatory reactions at the injection site and an unpleasant taste in the mouth. Contra-indications are pregnancy and breast-feeding, since calcitonin may inhibit lactation.

Alendronate increased BMD by about 4% in one year in a trial in Crohn's disease,[636] but while neither this nor any other treatment has yet been shown to reduce the incidence of fractures in patients with IBD, benefits are likely to be similar to those seen in coeliac disease.[133] However, it has been argued that the use of bisphosphonates should be restricted to patients with multiple risk factors for fractures, since the annual risk of a hip fracture in IBD patients less than 40 years old is only 0.04%.[621] Younger patients should therefore invoke lifestyle measures, proceeding to bisphosphonates only when reaching the age of 60, when the annual fracture risk rises to over 1%.[621]

BMD should be monitored yearly in patients on treatment. If BMD falls by more than 4% per year in two successive years another drug should be tried.[133,637] Bisphosphonate therapy deemed successful on BMD measurements should be continued for at least three years and if stopped, BMD measured again after one year. If BMD falls by more than 4%, treatment should be reinstituted.[133]

Haematology

Anaemia

Introduction. Mild anaemia (haemoglobin >10.5 g/dl) occurs in about one-third of patients with Crohn's disease.[638] Its causes include deficiencies of iron, vitamin B_{12} (in patients with terminal ileal disease or resection) and folate (due to increased cell turnover or extensive small bowel disease or resection) as well as cytokine-driven chronic inflammatory disease with a relative deficiency of erythropoietin.[638] Correction of all types of anaemia is an important aspect of the treatment of Crohn's since even when not severe, anaemia adversely affects cognitive function, ability to work and general well-being. Consequently, its effective treatment can make a substantial difference to quality of life.

While diagnosis and treatment of vitamin B_{12} and folate deficiency are straightforward (Figure 9.8), the same is not true of anaemia due to iron deficiency and/or chronic inflammation.

Iron deficiency anaemia. Causes and investigation: Iron deficiency in IBD is multi-factorial. Causes include reduced dietary intake, blood loss from inflamed mucosa, impaired absorption due to small intestinal inflammation[639] and, in some patients, extensive bowel resection.

Confirmation that microcytic anaemia in a patient with Crohn's disease is due to iron deficiency is not always easy. In patients without chronic inflammation, a reduced serum ferritin concentration is a reliable guide to iron stores but, as an acute phase protein, ferritin is frequently elevated despite co-existent iron deficiency in patients with active IBD. Similarly, iron and total iron-binding capacity (TIBC) levels are difficult to interpret in the presence of inflammation.[640] The serum transferrin receptor assay may prove useful in this situation[640] but is not yet widely available. The gold standard, bone marrow aspiration, stained for iron, is rarely used as it is invasive and unpleasant for the patient.

Management: Most patients with moderate iron deficiency respond satisfactorily to oral iron therapy (Figure 9.8). There is no good evidence to support

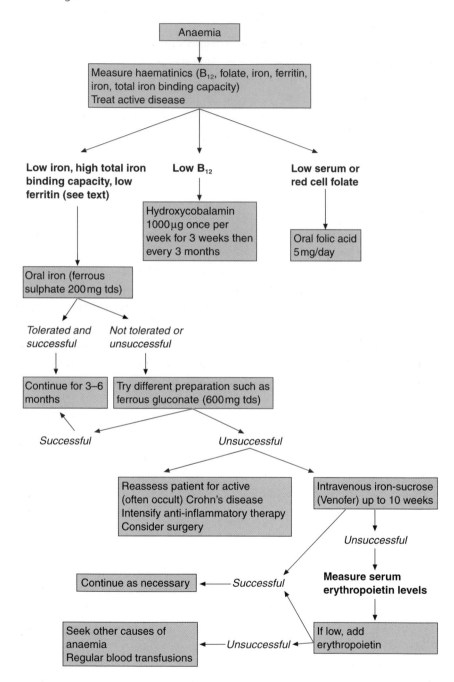

Figure 9.8 *Treatment of anaemia.*

the widely quoted view that such therapy is less well tolerated in patients with IBD than other non-inflammatory causes of anaemia.[641]

In about 15% of patients with Crohn's disease, the anaemia is more severe (haemoglobin <10.5 g/dl).[638] In patients not responding adequately to oral iron, intravenous iron-sucrose (Venofer) is efficacious and safe, two-thirds of patients responding within four weeks.[638,642] In the small minority of patients refractory to iron-sucrose infusions, supplemental erythropoietin (although expensive) can give good results, particularly if initial serum erythropoietin, transferrin and soluble transferrin levels are raised.[642–644]

Coagulopathy – arterial and venous thrombosis

Incidence and causes. Since the 1930s, clinical series have shown an increased incidence of arterial and venous thromboembolic disease in patients with IBD, ranging from 1 to 8%.[645] Autopsy studies indicate that underdiagnosis in life is common and that the true incidence may be higher (7–41%).[646,647]

Thromboembolism in Crohn's may occur at an unusually young age and in unusual sites such as the cerebral, mesenteric and hepatic arteries and veins; it is more common in relapse than remission.

Many patients have classical risk factors such as fluid depletion, immobility due to illness or operation, smoking or sepsis. Abnormal platelet function and coagulation are also relevant in patients with Crohn's. Thrombocytosis is common in active disease, and platelet activation and aggregation are increased.[648,649] Elevated levels of prothrombotic factor V Leiden mutation,[650] factor VIII and fibrinogen,[651] reduced levels of antithrombin III and protein S[652] and activated protein C resistance[653] may each play a part in some patients with thromboembolism.

Management. The prevention and treatment of thromboembolic complications of Crohn's resembles that for patients without the disease. Preventive measures include the avoidance and treatment of fluid depletion and sepsis, early mobilization, compression stockings and subcutaneous low dose heparin (Enoxaparin 20–40 mg/day).[395] Avoidance of smoking and oral contraceptives containing oestrogen is also advisable.[654]

Established venous and arterial thromboses are treated conventionally and apparently safely with intravenous heparin and warfarin. Caution is recommended if the use of thrombolytic therapy such as streptokinase is considered in patients with active Crohn's, because of the risks of bleeding from intestinal ulceration.

Psychosocial problems in Crohn's disease

Introduction

A recent meta-analysis has confirmed that quality of life in patients with Crohn's disease is worse than in patients with UC or controls; unsurprisingly quality of life varies inversely with disease activity.[113]

For a chronic condition with an uncertain outcome such as Crohn's disease, the global impact on individual patients can be influenced as much by psychosocial factors as by the physical symptoms themselves. Psychosocial symptoms, depression, anxiety and other mood disturbances may occur during exacerbations of disease and improve with remission of disease activity.[39] Recognition and management of these factors improve subjective sense of well-being and quality of life.[655] However, there is frequently a reluctance to discuss such issues during a doctor–patient consultation: this leads to needless 'suffering in silence' and a preoccupation with unexpressed concerns.[655]

Risk factors for psychological morbidity

The hypothesis that IBD occurs among patients of a particular psychological make-up has now been discounted (Chapter 1).[39] However, some patients with Crohn's disease are at special risk of developing psychological distress (Table 9.8). Some of the factors predisposing to psychological morbidity occur particularly at certain times during patients' lives, for example in relation to body image in adolescence.[656]

Several studies have suggested an increased lifetime risk of psychiatric illnesses in patients with Crohn's disease.[394] Both depression and anxiety are more common in Crohn's than UC, and predominate in the first year after diagnosis.[394] Psychiatric disturbances are particularly common in children with IBD (up to 60%);[657] indeed Crohn's disease in childhood may even present with psychiatric rather than physical symptoms.[658]

Patients' concerns about their illness and its impact on their life include a lack of energy; a lack of control over bowel habit; the effects of medications; the possibility of surgery or a stoma; their body image; social isolation; fear of unpredictable bouts of illness; the feeling of being a burden to partners, family and friends; feeling dirty; not reaching their full potential in education, employment, forming relationships or having a family and a lack of

Table 9.8 Risk factors for the development of psychological morbidity in Crohn's disease.[677]

Stress (daily versus major life events)
Symptom exacerbation
Comorbid psychiatric disorders (depression, anxiety)
Emotion-focused versus problem-focused coping
Lack of information about the disease and its course
Lack of social support
Inability to grieve over lost body image
Persistent anger or denial of illness
Feeling of loss of control
Social impairment

necessary information from the medical community.[655,656,659] Young patients are more likely to experience problems with interpersonal relationships, body image and physical concerns, while older patients are more likely to fear cancer.[656]

Management of psychological disturbance in Crohn's disease

Patients who seek help for psychosocial problems related to IBD tend to be female, with predominantly emotional and interpersonal problems.[660]

Education about IBD

Patients poorly informed about their disease tend to have the greatest concerns about it.[661] In a recent survey, 75% of patients attending medical clinics wanted more information and only 50% were aware of patients' associations such as the National Association for Colitis and Crohn's disease (NACC).[659] Whether more information about their disease alleviates patients' anxiety and improves their quality of life is uncertain.[662] Often, the IBD nurse (Chapter 10) is best placed to educate patients about Crohn's and discuss in depth disease-related concerns.

Counselling

Although its beneficial effects are difficult to prove, the availability of a counselling service is widely valued by patients. Counselling services are not widely available in the NHS and, as in other areas of deficiency (see below), the NACC has recently pioneered IBD-specific counselling in selected hospitals in the UK.

An early aim is to establish specific psychosocial problems and to ameliorate them as far as possible. A search for psychiatric illness is followed when necessary by referral to a psychiatrist with a special interest in chronic medical disorders.[663] Subsequent counselling measures range from supportive therapies to training in the use of cognitive coping mechanisms.

Medical therapies

Co-existing psychiatric morbidity needs to be treated appropriately.[394] Patients with depression, poor quality of life and high disease burden are more likely to attend their GP or gastroenterology clinic.[664] Addressing these problems may reduce their health care utilization as well as improve their general well-being.[664]

Social difficulties of patients with Crohn's disease

Whatever their ability to cope psychologically with Crohn's disease, patients face a variety of social difficulties.

Personal relationships and family life

Many patients with Crohn's disease experience on-going problems with ill-health, which can compromise interpersonal relationships.

Children may be reluctant to attend school, participate in sport or play with friends; some may become socially isolated.[665,666] These behavioural changes may in turn affect siblings. Parents of children with Crohn's feel that their work and family holidays are frequently disrupted.[665]

Adults may have problems with their marriage. Both marriage and divorce are more common in patients with Crohn's disease than in the general population.[667] The influence of Crohn's on sexual relationships, pregnancy and childbirth is covered in Chapter 7.

Schooling

Many children with Crohn's disease require time away from school, as a result of relapses with or without hospitalization.

In one case–control study, children with Crohn's disease had periods of two or more weeks off school more often than their peers (42% compared with 4%). However, their overall time away from school was lower than for controls.[668] Overall, 47% of children with Crohn's disease went on to further education, 17% had difficulties sitting exams and 14% did not feel that they had achieved their potential;[668] these figures were comparable with community controls.[666,669]

Booklets informing schoolteachers allow increased understanding of children's needs.[670,671] Equally, if examinations are taken during or shortly after times of illness, examining boards need to be notified; they may adjust gradings upwards, particularly if there is a discrepancy between results from course work and the examination itself.[666]

Work

Crohn's disease affects employment adversely, with proportionately more patients than controls off work and unemployed at a given time.[667,668] Symptom severity is twice as high for those unable to work, with inability to work being a marker of the global functional impact of the disease.[656] Patients with Crohn's disease are twice as likely to have a sedentary occupation.[667]

Employers' attitudes give cause for concern. A survey of personnel managers showed that up to 25% would not employ staff known to have IBD, and that 30% would not allow patients time off to attend outpatient appointments.[672] Perceived attitudes of employers mean that 20% of patients conceal their diagnosis of IBD.[666,673]

Life insurance

In patients with Crohn's disease, additional weightings are added to the standard premiums payable by the normal population for life, critical illness and permanent health insurance depending upon the perceived risks to the individual patient.[666,674] For example, the premiums may double or treble within one year of a major attack, decreasing between one and five years to standard levels by five years. After surgery, premiums return to normal beyond two years but may be weighted until this time, with features such as extracolonic disease and being undernourished adding additional weightings. Patients with dysplasia on colonic biopsies may find it difficult to obtain any cover at all.[674]

Role of self-help groups

Self-help groups are commonly formed by patients with chronic diseases which impact on multiple facets of their life.[675] The roles of groups such as the NACC (see Appendix) tend to reflect deficiencies in the provision of formal NHS health-care services.

At a national level, self-help groups provide information about Crohn's disease though pamphlets and websites (Chapters 6, 10 and Appendix), gather funds for research and act as a political pressure and reference group. Local subgroups provide opportunities for social and educational meetings, as well as informal advice and emotional support for patients and their relatives.[675]

Members of self-help groups such as the NACC clearly value their role.[675] It remains unclear, however, why only a minority (20–30%) of patients with IBD join a support group.[675] In some instances, at least, this is as a result of unawareness of their existence:[659] as indicated in Chapter 6, doctors and nurses seeing patients with IBD should make every effort to ensure they are given information about support groups such as NACC.

chapter 10

Management of Crohn's disease in the community and outpatient department

Introduction

This chapter discusses delivery of care for outpatients with Crohn's disease in the UK. Topics include the roles of general practitioners (GPs), hospital outpatient departments and specialist IBD nurses in the follow-up of patients in the community. The chapter concludes with a section about the costs of treating Crohn's disease.

Care of patients with Crohn's disease in general practice

The prevalence and incidence of Crohn's disease in the West (Table 1.1),[2] mean that in a British general practice population of 5000–7000 patients, there will be about five patients with Crohn's and one new patient diagnosed with Crohn's every two years. Inevitably, GPs' experience of managing Crohn's disease is limited, so that long-term follow-up is best co-ordinated primarily by a hospital-based specialist IBD service. There is, however, a place for guideline-directed shared care of patients with established Crohn's, and how this can be achieved is outlined below

The new patient with Crohn's disease

Delays in diagnosis of Crohn's are frequent[55,58] and may make the disease more complex in its pathology at diagnosis and more refractory to treatment. Additionally, delays in diagnosis may undermine patients' confidence in their doctors. The severity of many first attacks and the increased mortality associated with the first five years of diagnosis[71,72] make rapid diagnosis and treatment essential.[128]

The vast majority of patients presenting to their GP with diarrhoea and/or abdominal pain will have irritable bowel syndrome rather than Crohn's disease (or other serious disease) and it is a challenge to spot those who need prompt referral for further investigation. Pointers to a diagnosis of Crohn's disease are shown in Table 10.1.

Follow-up in general practice of patients with established Crohn's disease

Some patients with Crohn's disease, generally those with stable, inactive and limited disease, can be followed safely by their GP. This arrangement may be preferred by patients living far from their local hospital, but is dependent on appropriate shared-care guidelines as well as prompt open access to the hospital IBD clinic when necessary; such access is not always, unfortunately, available in the UK.[678,679]

Table 10.1 When to suspect Crohn's disease in general practice.

Symptoms	Diarrhoea (± blood) for >2 weeks, especially if nocturnal
	Persistent abdominal pain
	Weight loss
	Fever
	Complications (eyes, skin, joints, mouth ulcers)
	Family history of IBD
Signs	Systemic disturbance (fever, weight loss)
	Anaemia
	Abdominal tenderness or mass
	Perianal disease (fissure, fistula, abscess, tags, tenderness, induration)
Tests	Raised ESR, C-reactive protein, platelet count
	Anaemia
	Low albumin
	Negative stool culture

Many patients with Crohn's disease, unlike UC, however, are unsuitable for community-based follow-up and need to be seen regularly in a specialist hospital clinic (see below). Such patients include those with frequent relapses, corticosteroid or immunosuppressant-dependent disease, multiple previous operations, nutritional problems, growth failure, systemic complications or perianal sepsis.[680]

Patients with quiescent uncomplicated Crohn's who are suitable for follow-up by their GP need to have the frequency of review and investigation tailored according to the details of their disease. Review should include evaluation of current symptoms, weight and a blood test to check for disease activity and complications (Tables 10.2 and 10.3). Further blood tests may also be needed in patients on particular therapies (Table 10.2). Treatment should be reviewed at every visit and care taken to avoid inessential prescription of drugs, such as NSAIDs, which may exacerbate Crohn's disease.

Patients should be re-referred promptly to the hospital IBD clinic in the event of deterioration in their symptoms since, unlike UC, it cannot safely

Table 10.2 Investigations to monitor drug side effects.

Drug	Monitoring
Corticosteroids	Blood pressure Serum or urine glucose Serum sodium and potassium levels (3 to 6 monthly) DEXA scanning (Table 10.3 and Figure 9.7)
5-ASA	Baseline FBC, serum urea and creatinine, LFT, folate Sulphasalazine – 3 monthly FBC, folate, serum urea and creatinine, LFT Mesalazine – 6–12 monthly serum urea and creatinine
Azathioprine, 6-mercaptopurine, mycophenolate	Baseline: FBC, LFT, TPMT activity/genotype (thiopurines only) FBC and LFT fortnightly for 2 months then every 2–3 months
Methotrexate	FBC and LFT fortnightly for 2 months then every 2–3 months Lung function tests, CXR if patient breathless Liver biopsy, particularly with a cumulative dose of 5 g and/or if transaminases rise

FBC, full blood count; LFT, liver function tests; CXR, chest X-ray; DEXA, dual energy X-ray absorptiometry; TPMT, thiopurine methyl-transferase.

Table 10.3 Long-term monitoring for intra- and extraintestinal manifestations and complications.

Disease activity	Monitoring
General disease activity	FBC (haemoglobin, white cells and platelets), ESR, CRP, albumin
Nutritional status	Annual FBC, albumin, folate, B_{12}, ferritin, calcium, magnesium Height, weight and body mass index
Liver disease	Annual liver function tests
Bone density	Check DEXA if: Prednisolene >10 g/lifetime or >1 g/6 months; Men >55 years; women at menopause or when first seen Fragility fracture Monitor DEXA yearly (see Figure 9.7)
Colorectal carcinoma screening	Colonoscopy and multiple biopsies 8–10 years after onset of Crohn's colitis to establish disease extent and exclude dysplasia Repeat colonoscopy every 2 years if extensive disease; annually if primary sclerosing cholangitis, family history of colorectal carcinoma, refractory disease or co-existing adenoma

FBC, full blood count; ESR, erythrocyte sedimentation rate; CRP, C-reactive protein; DEXA, dual energy X-ray absorptiometry.

be assumed that treatment with a 5-ASA or corticosteroids is necessarily appropriate (Chapter 6).

Lastly, patients with extensive Crohn's colitis should be referred after eight to ten years to the hospital IBD clinic for consideration of colorectal cancer screening (Table 10.3) (Chapter 9).

Although, in appropriate patients, care by GPs with open access hospital follow-up is preferred by both patients and GPs, and is cheaper than conventional hospital follow-up,[678] there has been insufficient long-term follow-up of this arrangement to ensure that complications of the disease and its treatment are kept to a minimum.

Hospital outpatient follow-up

Purpose of hospital follow-up

The purpose of hospital follow-up is to provide optimal care to outpatients with IBD. This includes not only expertise and facilities for diagnosing and treating Crohn's disease and its complications, but also the provision of educational resources and contacts with self-help groups such as the NACC. Additionally, outpatient services provide training opportunities for doctors, nurses and other health carers, as well as opportunities for audit and research.

Organization of hospital outpatients

IBD clinics should be multi-disciplinary. A joint medical/surgical clinic run by clinicians with a special interest in the medical and surgical management of Crohn's disease is essential; IBD nurse specialists, a stoma therapist and dietitian should also attend. In some clinics, an IBD-trained counsellor is also present (Chapter 9).

Staffing resources in outpatients should allow an unhurried consultation with 30 minutes for new patients and for their first re-attendance. Subsequent follow-up appointments can usually be completed in 10 minutes, although during an outpatient session there will inevitably be several patients requiring a longer time for review. Patients under long-term follow-up should be able to see a consultant promptly whenever necessary and at least at every third visit in order to maximize continuity of care and prevent deferring of management decisions.

Educational leaflets from patient support groups should be freely available in the clinic. There should be an adequate number of toilets of good quality.[128]

Monitoring of Crohn's disease and its treatment

Outpatient consultations should include a symptom review, examination as necessary and blood or other tests depending on the nature of the individual patient's disease and treatment (Tables 10.2 and 10.3) (Chapters 3, 6 and 9). Investigations should be undertaken and their results reviewed promptly, so that necessary changes in patient management can be expedited.

Self-treatment strategies

It has been suggested that, in patients with UC, provision of a strict protocol safely allows self-guided therapy in the event of relapse.[681] This strategy appears to reduce the number of follow-up appointments and allows more rapid access to the clinic by patients needing to be seen quickly. However, the symptoms of active Crohn's, and in particular its treatment, vary according to the location of the disease and the underlying pathology (Chapter 6). Self-treatment by patients with Crohn's may therefore, be inappropriate and worsen outcome.

IBD nurse

In other fields of medicine, for example diabetes, the usefulness of nurse specialists is well established. The post of IBD nurse is a more recent innovation which is making an increasing impact on patient care.[682]

Patient follow-up

The role of the IBD nurse specialist depends on local resources and needs. In many hospitals, the nurse runs a clinic in which he/she sees follow-up patients and, within agreed guidelines, recommends treatment or immediate review by a doctor.

Additionally, the nurse is often well placed to field telephone calls from IBD patients. Many routine enquiries can be solved over the telephone, while others require triage.[682] A recent audit found that the appointment of an IBD nurse was followed by a reduction in outpatient attendances, hospital admissions and total bed stays. Patient satisfaction was also increased, particularly in relation to information about IBD, access to doctors when needed and emotional support.[683]

Education

A major role of the IBD nurse is to educate patients and their families about IBD.[683] Education is best managed by personal interviews with newly diagnosed patients and by provision of information sheets. The educational value of the IBD nurse extends further: depending on local circumstances, he/she can usefully hold information sessions with GPs, other nurses and representatives of pharmaceutical companies.

Other roles

Other roles of the IBD nurse will depend on the requirements of the hospital. They include maintaining IBD patient databases, undertaking audit, co-ordinating clinical trials and providing a flexible sigmoidoscopy service.

Conclusion

As Nightingale concludes,[682] the IBD nurse plays a key role in improving education, satisfaction and management of patients with Crohn's disease. Every hospital should have one.

Health economics and the costs of Crohn's disease

The costs associated with any disease are direct and indirect.[684–686] Direct costs comprise those incurred by the health-care services as a result of providing treatment. Indirect costs arise from the impact of the disease on the patient's social, economic and physical well-being, and are greater and even more difficult to assess than direct costs.[686]

In studies of 100 patients with Crohn's disease,[687,688] the mean annual direct costs of the disease in the USA in 1990 were about $6500 (£4000) per patient. Hospital admissions and surgery accounted for nearly 80% of the costs, drugs 11%, investigations and outpatient attendances 5% and the management of extraintestinal complications 5%. About 20% of the patient population generated 80% of the health costs: the annual direct costs of these individuals were about $26 000 (£16 000) per patient. Reworking of these sums to 1996 figures[685] produced estimates of $9200 (£5800) for mean annual direct costs for all Crohn's disease patients, and $37 000 (£23 000) for the sickest 20%. There are unfortunately no strong data about the UK costs of managing Crohn's disease.

As indicated above, the costs of managing individual patients or groups of patients with Crohn's disease depend on a range of factors which include disease phenotype, drugs used and the need for hospital admission and/or surgery. Data on some of these variables already exist,[235,689–692] and the introduction of expensive biological therapies such as infliximab has stimulated further studies.[684,685]

In assessing the economic impact of a new therapy such as infliximab, it is essential to consider not only prescribing costs, but also the positive economic effects of improving clinical outcomes. In particular, if a new agent reduces the need for hospital admission and surgery, its net direct costs would be substantially reduced. Similarly, by restoring sick patients' ability to work, and/or productivity there, a new agent could reduce the indirect costs of Crohn's. Full reports on the magnitude of these effects for new treatments such as infliximab are not yet available.

References

1. Shivananda S, Lennard-Jones J, Logan R et al. Incidence of inflammatory bowel disease across Europe: is there a difference between north and south? Results of the European Collaborative Study on Inflammatory Bowel Disease. *Gut* 1996; **39**: 690–7.

2. Loftus EV Jr, Schoenfeld P, Sandborn WJ. The epidemiology and natural history of Crohn's disease in population-based patient cohorts from North America: a systematic review. *Aliment Pharmacol Ther* 2002; **16**: 51–60.

3. Gent AE, Hellier MD, Grace RH et al. Inflammatory bowel disease and domestic hygiene in infancy. *Lancet* 1994; **343**: 766–7.

4. Montgomery SM, Pounder RE, Wakefield AJ. Infant mortality and the incidence of inflammatory bowel disease. *Lancet* 1997; **349**: 472–3.

5. Feehally J, Burden AC, Mayberry JF et al. Disease variations in Asians in Leicester. *Q J Med* 1993; **86**: 263–9.

6. Shanahan F. Crohn's disease. *Lancet* 2002; **359**: 62–9.

7. Satsangi J, Grootscholten C, Holt H et al. Clinical patterns of familial inflammatory bowel disease. *Gut* 1996; **38**: 738–41.

8. Tysk C, Lindberg E, Jarnerot G et al. Ulcerative colitis and Crohn's disease in an unselected population of monozygotic and dizygotic twins. A study of heritability and the influence of smoking. *Gut* 1988; **29**: 990–6.

9. Hugot JP, Chamaillard M, Zouali H et al. Association of NOD2 leucine-rich repeat variants with susceptibility to Crohn's disease. *Nature* 2001; **411**: 599–603.

10. McGovern DP, van Heel DA, Ahmad T et al. NOD2 (CARD15), the first susceptibility gene for Crohn's disease. *Gut* 2001; **49**: 752–4.

11. Rioux JD, Daly MJ, Silverberg MS et al. Genetic variation in the 5q31 cytokine gene cluster confers susceptibility to Crohn disease. *Nat Genet* 2001; **29**: 223–8.

12. Ogura Y, Bonen DK, Inohara N et al. A frameshift mutation in NOD2 associated with susceptibility to Crohn's disease. *Nature* 2001; **411**: 603–6.

13. Ahmad T, Armuzzi A, Bunce M et al. The molecular classification of the clinical manifestations of Crohn's disease. *Gastroenterology* 2002; **122**: 854–66.

14. Hampe J, Grebe J, Nikolaus S et al. Association of NOD 2 (CARD 15) genotype with clinical course of Crohn's disease: a cohort study. *Lancet* 2002; **359**: 1661–5.

15. Elson CO. Genes, microbes, and T-cells–new therapeutic targets in Crohn's disease. *N Engl J Med* 2002; **346**: 614–16.

16. Shanahan F. Antibody 'markers' in Crohn's disease: opportunity or overstatement? *Gut* 1997; **40**: 557–8.

17. Shanahan F. Inflammatory bowel disease: immunodiagnostics, immunothera-peutics, and ecotherapeutics. *Gastroenterology* 2001; **120**: 622–35.
18. Sutton CL, Yang H, Rotter J et al. Familial expression of anti-*Saccharomyces cervisiae mannan* antibodies in affected and unaffected relatives of patients with Crohn's disease. *Gut* 2000; **46**: 58–63.
19. Vasiliauskas EA, Kam LY, Karp LC et al. Marker antibody expression stratifies Crohn' disease into immunologically homogenous subgroups with distinct clinical characteristics. *Gut* 2000; **47**: 487–96.
20. Cope GF, Heatley RV. Cigarette smoking and intestinal defences. *Gut* 1992; **33**: 721–3.
21. Bridger S, Lee JCW, Bjarnason I et al. In siblings with similar genetic susceptibility for inflammatory bowel disease, smokers tend to develop Crohn's disease and non-smokers develop ulcerative colitis. *Gut* 2002; **51**: 21–5.
22. Sutherland LR, Ramcharan S, Bryant H et al. Effect of cigarette smoking on recurrence of Crohn's disease. *Gastroenterology* 1990; **98**: 1123–8.
23. Cottone M, Rosselli M, Orlando A et al. Smoking habits and recurrence in Crohn's disease. *Gastroenterology* 1994; **106**: 643–8.
24. Cosnes J, Beaugerie L, Carbonnel F et al. Smoking cessation and the course of Crohn's disease: an intervention study. *Gastroenterology* 2001; **120**: 1093–9.
25. Fernandez-Benares F, Cabre E, Esteve-Comas M et al. How effective is enteral nutrition in inducing clinical remission in Crohn's disease? A meta-analysis of the randomised clinical results. *J Parenter Enteral Nutr* 1995; **19**: 356–64.
26. Griffiths AM, Ohlsson A, Scherman PM et al. Meta-analysis of enteral nutrition as a primary treatment of active Crohn's disease. *Gastroenterology* 1995; **108**: 1056–67.
27. Riordan AM, Hunter JO, Cowan RE et al. Treatment of active Crohn's disease by exclusion diet: East Anglian multicentre controlled trial. *Lancet* 1993; **342**: 1131–4.
28. Reif S, Klein I, Lubin F et al. Pre-illness dietary factors in inflammatory bowel disease. *Gut* 1997; **40**: 754–60.
29. Powell JJ, Harvey RS, Ashwood P et al. Immune potentiation of ultrafine dietary particles in normal subjects and patients with inflammatory bowel disease. *J Autoimmun* 2000; **14**: 99–105.
30. Hermon-Taylor J. *Mycobacterium avium* subspecies *paratuberculosis* in the causation of Crohn's disease. *World J Gastroenterol* 2000; **6**: 630–2.
31. Wakefield AJ, Ekbom AM, Dhillon AP et al. Crohn's disease: pathogenesis and persistent measles infection. *Gastroenterology* 1995; **108**: 911–16.
32. Ghosh S, Armitage E, Wilson D et al. Detection of persistent measles virus infection in Crohn's disease: current state of experimental work. *Gut* 2001; **48**: 748–52.
33. Shanahan F. Probiotics and inflammatory bowel disease: is there a scientific rationale? *Inflamm Bowel Dis* 2000; **6**: 107–15.
34. Bjarnason I, Hayllar J, MacPherson AJ et al. Side effects of non steroidal anti-inflammatory drugs in small and large intestine in humans. *Gastroenterology* 1993; **104**: 1832–47.
35. Wallace JL. Prostaglandin biology in inflammatory bowel disease. *Gastroenterol Clin North Am* 2001; **30**: 971–80.
36. Bonner GF. Using Cox-2 inhibitors in IBD: anti-inflammatories inflame a controversy. *Am J Gastroenterol* 2002; **97**: 783–4.
37. Demling L. Is Crohn's disease caused by antibiotics? *Hepatogastroenterology* 1994; **41**: 549–51.
38. Boyko EJ, Theis MK, Vaughan TL et al. Increased risk of inflammatory bowel disease associated with oral contraceptive use. *Am J Epidemiol* 1994; **140**: 268–78.

39. Porcelli P, Leoci C, Guerra V. A prospective study of the relationship between disease activity and psychologic distress in patients with inflammatory bowel disease. *Scand J Gastroenterol* 1996; **31**: 792–6.
40. Barrett SM, Standen PJ, Lee AS et al. Personality, smoking and inflammatory bowel disease. *Eur J Gastroenterol Hepatol* 1996; **8**: 651–6.
41. North CS, Alpers DH. A review of studies of psychiatric factors in Crohn's disease: etiologic implications. *Ann Clin Psychiatry* 1994; **6**: 117–24.
42. Qiu BS, Vallance BA, Blennerhassett PA et al. The role of CD4+ lymphocytes in the susceptibility of mice to stress-induced reactivation of experimental colitis. *Nature Med* 1999; **5**: 1178–82.
43. North CS, Alpers DH, Helzer JE et al. Do life events or depression exacerbate inflammatory bowel disease? A prospective study. *Ann Intern Med* 1991; **114**: 381–6.
44. von Wietersheim J, Kohler T, Feiereis H. Relapse-precipitating life events and feelings in patients with inflammatory bowel disease. *Psychother Psychosom* 1992; **58**: 103–12.
45. Papadakis KA, Targan SR. Role of cytokines in the pathogenesis of inflammatory bowel disease. *Annu Rev Med* 2000; **51**: 289–98.
46. Fiocchi C. Inflammatory bowel disease: etiology and pathogenesis. *Gastroenterology* 1998; **115**: 182–205.
47. Nikolaus S, Raedler A, Kuhbacker T et al. Mechanisms in failure of infliximab for Crohn's disease. *Lancet* 2000; **356**: 1475–9.
48. van Deventer SJH. Small therapeutic molecules for the treatment of inflammatory bowel disease. *Gut* 2002; **50**(Suppl 3): 47–53.
49. Simmonds NJ, Rampton DS. Inflammatory bowel disease – a radical view. *Gut* 1993; **34**: 865–8.
50. Kubes P. Inducible nitric oxide synthase: a little bit of good in all of us. *Gut* 2000; **47**: 6–9.
51. Schuppan D, Hahn EG. MMPs in the gut: inflammation hits the matrix. *Gut* 2000; **47**: 12–14.
52. Wyatt J, Vogelsang H, Hubl W et al. Intestinal permeability and the prediction of relapse in Crohn's disease. *Lancet* 1993; **341**: 1437–9.
53. Collins CE. Rampton DS. Review article: platelets in inflammatory bowel disease – pathogenic role and therapeutic implications. *Aliment Pharmacol Ther* 1997; **11**: 237–47.
54. Wakefield AL, Sawyerr AM, Dhillon AP et al. Pathogenesis of Crohn's disease: multifocal gastrointestinal infarction. *Lancet* 1989; **ii**: 1057–62.
55. Farmer RG, Hawk WA, Turnbull RB Jr. Clinical patterns in Crohn's disease: a statistical study of 615 cases. *Gastroenterology* 1975; **68**: 627–35.
56. Lapidus A, Bernell O, Hellers G et al. Clinical course of colorectal Crohn's disease: a 35 year follow-up study of 507 patients. *Gastroenterology* 1998; **114**: 1151–60.
57. Meyers S, Janowitz HD. 'Natural history' of Crohn's disease. An analytical review of the placebo lesson. *Gastroenterology* 1984; **87**: 1189–92.
58. Lapidus A, Bernell O, Hellers G et al. Incidence of Crohn's disease in Stockholm County 1955–1989. *Gut* 1997; **41**: 480–6.
59. McKee RF, Keenan RA. Perianal Crohn's disease—is it all bad news? *Dis Colon Rectum* 1996; **39**: 136–42.
60. Decker GA, Loftus EV Jr, Pasha TM et al. Crohn's disease of the esophagus: clinical features and outcomes. *Inflamm Bowel Dis* 2001; **7**: 113–19.
61. Yamamoto T, Allan RN, Keighley MR. An audit of gastroduodenal Crohn's disease: clinicopathologic features and management. *Scand J Gastroenterol* 1999; **34**: 1019–24.
62. Williams AJ, Wray D, Ferguson A. The clinical entity of orofacial Crohn's disease. *Q J Med* 1991; **79**: 451–8.

63. Pittock S, Drumm B, Fleming P et al. The oral cavity in Crohn's disease. *J Pediatr* 2001; **138**: 767–71.
64. Eveson JW. Granulomatous disorders of the oral mucosa. *Semin Diagn Pathol* 1996; **13**: 118–27.
65. Binder V, Hendriken C, Kreiner S. Prognosis in Crohn's disease – based on results from a regional patient group from the county of Copenhagen. *Gut* 1985; **26**: 146–50.
66. Gasche C, Scholmerich J, Brynskov J et al. A simple classification of Crohn's disease: report for the Working Party for the World Congresses of Gastroenterology, Vienna 1998. *Inflamm Bowel Dis* 2000; **6**: 8–15.
67. Lock MR, Farmer RG, Fazio VW et al. Recurrence and reoperation for Crohn's disease: the role of disease location in prognosis. *N Engl J Med* 1981; **304**: 1586–8.
68. Farmer RG, Whelan G, Fazio VW. Long-term follow-up of patients with Crohn's disease. Relationship between clinical pattern and prognosis. *Gastroenterology* 1985; **88**: 1818–25.
69. Polito JM, Childs B, Mellits ED et al. Crohn's disease: influence of age at diagnosis on site and clinical type of disease. *Gastroenterology* 1996; **111**: 580–6.
70. Rioux JD, Silverberg MS, Daly MJ et al. Genomewide search in Canadian families with inflammatory bowel disease reveals two novel susceptibility loci. *Am J Hum Genet* 2000; **66**: 1863–70.
71. Probert CS, Jayanthi V, Wicks AC et al. Mortality from Crohn's disease in Leicestershire, 1972–1989: an epidemiological community based study. *Gut* 1992; **33**: 1226–8.
72. Munkholm P, Langholz E, Davidsen E, Binder V. Intestinal cancer risk and mortality in patients with Crohn's disease. *Gastroenterology* 1993; **105**: 1716–23.
73. Jess T, Winther KV, Munkholm P et al. Mortality and causes of death in Crohn's disease: follow up of a population-based cohort in Copenhagen County, Denmark. *Gastroenterology* 2002; **122**: 1808–14.
74. Ekbom A, Helmick CG, Zack M et al. Survival and causes of death in patients with inflammatory bowel disease: a population-based study. *Gastroenterology* 1992; **103**: 954–60.
75. Bebb JR, Logan RP. Review article: does the use of immunosuppressive therapy in inflammatory bowel disease increase the risk of developing lymphoma? *Aliment Pharmacol Ther* 2001; **8**: 93–7.
76. Hodgson HJF. Laboratory markers of inflammatory bowel disease. In: Allan RN, Rhodes JM, Hanauer SB et al, eds. *Inflammatory bowel diseases*, 3rd ed. New York: Churchill Livingstone, 1997, 329–34.
77. Sendid B, Colombel JF, Jacquinot PM et al. Specific antibody response to oligomannosidic epitopes in Crohn's disease. *Clin Diagn Lab Immunol* 1996; **3**: 219–26.
78. Pulimood AB, Ramakrishna BS, Kurian G et al. Endoscopic mucosal biopsies are useful in distinguishing granulomatous colitis due to Crohn's disease from tuberculosis. *Gut* 1999; **45**: 537–41.
79. Gan HT, Chan YQ, Onyang Q et al. Differentiation between intestinal tuberculosis and Crohn's disease in endoscopic biopsies by polymerase chain reaction. *Am J Gastroenterol* 2002; **97**: 1446–51.
80. Cellier C, Sahmoud T, Froguel et al. Correlations between clinical activity, endoscopic severity, and biological parameters in colonic or ileocolonic Crohn's disease. A prospective multicentre study of 121 cases. Groupe d'Etude Therapeutique des Affections Inflammatoires Digestives. *Gut* 1994; **35**: 231–5.
81. Friedman S, Rubin PH, Bodian C et al. Screening and surveillance colonoscopy in chronic Crohn's colitis. *Gastroenterology* 2001; **120**: 820–6.

82. Rutgeerts P, Geboes K, Vantrappen G et al. Predictability of the postoperative course of Crohn's disease. *Gastroenterology* 1990; **99**: 956–63.

83. Iddan G, Meron G, Glukhovsky A et al. Wireless capsule endoscopy. *Nature* 2000; **405**: 417.

84. Warren BF. Histopathology: central to the diagnosis and management of inflammatory bowel disease. In: Rampton DS, ed. *Inflammatory Bowel Disease, Clinical Diagnosis and Management.* London: Martin Dunitz Ltd, 2000, 87–105.

85. Bartram CI. Radiology in the current assessment of ulcerative colitis. *Gastrointest Radiol* 1977; **25**: 383–92.

86. Wills JS, Lobis IF, Denstman FJ. Crohn's disease: state of the art. *Radiology* 1997; **202**: 597–610.

87. Gasche C, Schober E, Turetschek K. Small bowel barium studies in Crohn's disease. *Gastroenterology* 1998; **114**: 1349.

88. Giaffer MH. Labelled leucocyte scintigraphy in inflammatory bowel disease: clinical applications. *Gut* 1996; **38**: 1–5.

89. Gibson P, Lichtenstein M, Salehi N et al. Value of positive technetium-99m leucocyte scans in predicting intestinal inflammation. *Gut* 1991; **32**: 1502–7.

90. Nyhlin H, Merrick MV, Eastwood MA. Bile acid malabsorption in Crohn's disease and indications for its assessment using SeHCAT. *Gut* 1994; **35**: 90–3.

91. Parente F, Maconi G, Bollani S. Bowel ultrasound in assessment of Crohn's disease and detection of related small bowel strictures: a prospective comparative study versus x-ray and intraoperative findings. *Gut* 2002; **50**: 490–5.

92. Schwartz DA, Wiersema MJ, Dudiak KM et al. A comparison of endoscopic ultrasound, magnetic resonance imaging, and examination under anesthesia for evaluation of Crohn's perianal fistulas. *Gastroenterology* 2001; **121**: 1064–72.

93. Low RN, Francis IR. MR imaging of the gastrointestinal tract with i.v. gadolinium and diluted barium oral contrast media compared with unenhanced MR imaging and CT. *Am J Roentgenol* 1997; **169**: 31–5.

94. Shoenut JP, Semelka RC, Magro CM et al. Comparison of magnetic resonance imaging and endoscopy in distinguishing the type and severity of inflammatory bowel disease. *J Clin Gastroenterol* 1994; **19**: 31–5.

95. Bicik I, Bauerfeind P, Breitbach T et al. Inflammatory bowel disease activity measured by positron-emission tomography. *Lancet* 1997; **350**: 262.

96. Kjeldsen J, Schaffalitzky de Muckadell OB. Assessment of disease severity and activity in inflammatory bowel disease. *Scand J Gastroenterol* 1993; **28**: 1–9.

97. Best WR, Becktel JM, Singleton JW et al. Development of a Crohn's disease activity index. *Gastroenterology* 1976; **70**: 439–44.

98. Harvey RF, Bradshaw JM. A simple index of Crohn's disease activity. *Lancet* 1980; **i**: 514.

99. Rampton DS, Shanahan F. *Inflammatory Bowel Disease.* Fast Facts Series. Oxford: Health Press, 2000.

100. Rampton DS. Management of Crohn's disease. *Br Med J* 1999; **319**: 1480–5.

101. Lim AG. What is the differential diagnosis of IBD? In: Rampton DS, ed. *Inflammatory Bowel Disease, Clinical Diagnosis and Management.* London: Martin Dunitz Ltd, 2000, 71–85.

102. Sartor RB. Review article: How relevant to human inflammatory bowel disease are current animal models of intestinal inflammation? *Aliment Pharmacol Ther* 1997; **11**(Suppl 3): 89–96.

103. Feagan BG, McDonald JW, Koval JJ. Therapeutics and inflammatory bowel disease: a guide to the interpretation of randomised controlled trials. *Gastroenterology* 1996; **110**: 275–83.

104. Sandborn WJ, Targan SR. Biologic therapy of inflammatory bowel disease. *Gastroenterology* 2002; **122**: 1592–608.

105. Carty E, Rampton DS. Evaluating novel therapies in inflammatory bowel disease. *Br J Clin Pharmacol* 2003; in press.
106. Brzinski A, Lashener BA. Natural history of Crohn's disease. In: Allan RN, Rhodes JM, Hanauer SB et al, eds. *Inflammatory Bowel Diseases*, 3rd ed. New York: Churchill Livingstone, 1997, 475–86.
107. Nugent SG, Kumar D, Rampton DS et al. Intestinal luminal pH in inflammatory bowel disease: possible determinants and implications for therapy with amino-salicylates and other drugs. *Gut* 2001; **48**: 571–7.
108. Taylor KD, Plevy SE, Yang H et al. ANCA pattern and LTA haplotype relationship to clinical responses to anti-TNF antibody treatment in Crohn's disease. *Gastroenterology* 2001; **120**: 1347–55.
109. Esters N, Vermeire S, Joossens S et al. Serological markers for prediction of response to anti-TNF treatment in Crohn's disease. *Am J Gastroenterol* 2002; **97**: 1458–62.
110. Tremaine WJ. Failure to yield: drug resistance in inflammatory bowel disease. *Gastroenterology* 2002; **122**: 1165–7.
111. Sandborn WJ, Feagan BG, Hanauer SB et al. A review of activity indices and efficacy endpoints for clinical trials of medical therapy in adults with Crohn's disease. *Gastroenterology* 2002; **122**: 512–30.
112. Irvine EJ, Feagan B, Rochon J et al. Quality of life: a valid and reliable measure of therapeutic efficacy in the treatment of inflammatory bowel disease. *Gastroenterology* 1994; **106**: 287–96.
113. Cohen RD. The quality of life in patients with Crohn's disease. *Aliment Pharmacol Ther* 2002; **16**: 1603–9.
114. Present DH, Korelitz BI, Wisch N et al. Treatment of Crohn's disease with 6-mercaptopurine. A long-term, randomized, double-blind study. *N Engl J Med* 1980; **302**: 981–7.
115. Present DH, Rutgeerts P, Targan S et al. Infliximab for the treatment of fistulas in patients with Crohn's disease. *N Engl J Med* 1999; **340**: 1398–1405.
116. Savarymuttu SH, Peters AM, Hodgson HJ, Chadwick VS. Assessment of disease activity in ulcerative colitis using indium-111-labelled leukocyte faecal excretion. *Scand J Gastroenterol* 1983; **18**: 907–12.
117. Tibble JA, Sigthorsson G, Bridger S et al. Surrogate markers of intestinal inflammation are predictive of relapse in patients with inflammatory bowel disease. *Gastroenterology* 2000; **119**: 15–22.
118. Modigliani R, Mary JY, Simon JF et al. Clinical, biological, and endoscopic picture of attacks of Crohn's disease. Evolution on prednisolone. Groupe d'Etude Therapeutique des Affections Inflammatoires Digestives. *Gastroenterology* 1990; **98**: 811–18.
119. D'Haens G, Geboes K, Ponette E et al. Healing of severe recurrent ileitis with azathioprine therapy in patients with Crohn's disease. *Gastroenterology* 1997; **112**: 1475–81.
120. D'Haens G, van Deventer S, van Hogezand R et al. Endoscopic and histological healing with infliximab anti-tumor necrosis factor antibodies in Crohn's disease: a European multicenter trial. *Gastroenterology* 1999; **116**: 1029–34.
121. Barnes PJ. Therapeutic strategies for allergic diseases. *Nature* 1999; **402** (6760 Suppl): B31–8.
122. Hanauer SB, Sandborn W. Management of Crohn's disease in adults. *Am J Gastroenterol* 2001; **96**: 635–43.
123. Greenberg GR, Feagan BG, Martin F et al. Oral budesonide for active Crohn's disease. *N Engl J Med* 1994; **331**: 836–41.
124. Rutgeerts P, Lofberg R, Malchow H et al. A comparison of budesonide with prednisolone for active Crohn's disease. *N Engl J Med* 1994; **331**: 842–5.

125. Thomsen OO, Cortot A, Jewell D et al. A comparison of budesonide and mesalamine for active Crohn's disease. International Budesonide–Mesalamine Study Group. *N Engl J Med* 1998; **339**: 370–4.
126. Papi C, Luchetti R, Gili L et al. Budesonide in the treatment of Crohn's disease: a meta-analysis. *Aliment Pharmacol Ther* 2000; **14**: 1419–28.
127. Summers RW, Switz DM, Sessions JT et al. National co-operative Crohn's disease study: results of drug treatment. *Gastroenterology* 1979; **77**: 847–69.
128. British Society of Gastroenterology. *Guidelines for the Management of Inflammatory Bowel Disease* 2003. In preparation.
129. Faubion WA Jr, Loftus EV Jr, Harmsen WS et al. The natural history of corticosteroid therapy for inflammatory bowel disease: a population-based study. *Gastroenterology* 2001; **121**: 255–60.
130. Farrell RJ, Murphy A, Long A et al. High multidrug resistance (P-glycoprotein 170) expression in inflammatory bowel disease who fail medical therapy. *Gastroenterology* 2000; **118**: 279–88.
131. Greenberg GR, Feagan BG, Martin F et al. Oral budesonide as maintenance treatment for Crohn's disease: a placebo-controlled, dose-ranging study. *Gastroenterology* 1996; **110**: 45–51.
132. Löfberg R, Rutgeerts P, Malchow H et al. Budesonide prolongs time to relapse in ileal and ileocaecal Crohn's disease. A placebo controlled one year study. *Gut* 1996; **39**: 82–6.
133. Scott EM, Gaywood I, Scott BB. Guidelines for osteoporosis in coeliac disease and inflammatory bowel disease. *Gut* 2000; **46**(Suppl 1): I1–8.
134. Munkholm P, Langholz E, Davidsen E et al. Frequency of glucocorticoid resistance and dependency in Crohn's disease. *Gut* 1994; **35**: 360–2.
135. Rutgeerts PJ. Review article: the limitations of corticosteroid therapy in Crohn's disease. *Aliment Pharmacol Ther* 2001; **15**: 1515–25.
136. Gelbmann CM, Rogler G, Gross V et al. Prior bowel resections, perianal disease, and a high initial Crohn's disease activity index are associated with corticosteroid resistance in active Crohn's disease. *Am J Gastroenterol* 2002; **97**: 1438–45.
137. Hanauer SB. Drug therapy: inflammatory bowel disease. *N Engl J Med* 1996; **334**: 841–8.
138. Sutherland LR. Sulphasalazine and the new salicylates. In: Allan RN, Rhodes JM, Hanauer SB et al. eds. *Inflammatory Bowel Diseases*, 3rd ed. New York: Churchill Livingstone, 1997, 487–502.
139. Singleton JW, Hanauer SB, Gitnick GL et al. Mesalamine capsules for the treatment of active Crohn's disease: results of a 16-week trial. *Gastroenterology* 1993; **104**: 1293–301.
140. Tremaine WJ, Schroeder KW, Harrison JM et al. A randomised, double-blind placebo controlled trial of the oral mesalamine (5-ASA) preparation, Asacol, in the treatment of symptomatic Crohn's colitis and ileocolitis. *J Clin Gastroenterol* 1994; **19**: 278–82.
141. Prantera C, Cottone M, Pallone F et al. Mesalamine in the treatment of mild and moderate active Crohn's ileitis: results of a randomized, multicenter trial. *Gastroenterology* 1999; **116**: 521–6.
142. Cammá C, Giunta M, Rosselli M et al. Mesalazine in the maintenance treatment of Crohn's disease: a meta-analysis adjusted for confounding variables. *Gastroenterology* 1997; **113**: 1465–73.
143. Lochs H, Mayer M, Fleig WE et al. Prophylaxis of postoperative relapse in Crohn's disease with mesalamine: European Cooperative Crohn's disease Study VI. *Gastroenterology* 2000; **118**: 264–73.
144. Sutherland LR. Mesalamine for the prevention of postoperative recurrence: is nearly there the same as being there? *Gastroenterology* 2000; **118**: 436–8.

145. Sutherland LR. Mesalamine and relapse prevention in Crohn's disease. *Gastroenterology* 2000; **118**: 597.

146. Anonymous. Blood dyscrasias and mesalazine. *Curr Prob Pharmacovig* 2000; **21**: 5.

147. World MJ, Stevens PE, Ashton MA et al. Mesalazine-associated interstitial nephritis. *Nephrology, Dialysis and Transplantation* 1996; **11**: 614–21.

148. Lowry PW, Franklin CL, Weaver AL et al. Leucopenia resulting from a drug interaction between azathioprine or 6-mercaptopurine and mesalamine, sulphasalazine, or balsalazide. *Gut* 2001; **49**: 656–64.

149. Dewit O, Vanheurverzwyn R, Desager JP et al. Interaction between azathioprine and aminosalicylates: an in vivo study in patients with Crohn's disease. *Aliment Pharmacol Ther* 2002; **16**: 79–85.

150. Wandall JH, Binder V. Leucocyte function in Crohn's disease. Studies on mobilisation using a quantitative skin window technique and on the function of circulating polymorphonuclear leucocytes in vitro. *Gut* 1982; **23**: 173–80.

151. Ursing B, Alm T, Barany F et al. A comparative study of metronidazole and sulphasalazine for active Crohn's disease: the Co-operative Crohn's disease study in Sweden II. Result. *Gastroenterology* 1982; **83**: 550–62.

152. Sutherland L, Singleton J, Sessions J et al. Double-blind, placebo controlled trial of metronidazole in Crohn's disease. *Gut* 1991; **32**: 1071–5.

153. Ambrose NS, Allan RN, Keighley MR et al. Antibiotic therapy for treatment in relapse of Crohn's disease. A prospective randomized study. *Dis Colon Rectum* 1985; **28**: 81–5.

154. Prantera C, Zannoni F, Scribano ML et al. An antibiotic regime for the treatment of active Crohn's disease: a randomized controlled clinical trial of metronidazole plus ciprofloxacin. *Am J Gastroenterol* 1996; **91**: 328–32.

155. Greenbloom SL, Steinhart AH, Greenberg GR. Combination ciprofloxacin and metronidazole for active Crohn's disease. *Can J Gastroenterol* 1998; **12**: 53–6.

156. Bernstein LH, Frank MS, Brandt LJ et al. Healing of perianal Crohn's disease with metronidazole. *Gastroenterology* 1980; **79**: 357–65.

157. Rutgeerts P, Hiele M, Geboes K et al. Controlled trial of metronidazole treatment for prevention of Crohn's recurrence after ileal resection. *Gastroenterology* 1995; **108**: 1617–21.

158. Duffy LF, Daum F, Fisher SE et al. Peripheral neuropathy in Crohn's disease patients treated with metronidazole. *Gastroenterology* 1985; **88**: 681–4.

159. Colombel JF, Lemann M, Cassagnou M et al. A controlled trial comparing ciprofloxacin with mesalazine for the treatment of active Crohn's disease. Groupe d'Etudes Therapeutiques des Affections Inflammatoires Digestives (GETAID). *Am J Gastroenterol* 1999; **94**: 674–8.

160. Arnold GL, Beaves MR, Pryjdun VO et al. Preliminary study of ciprofloxacin in active Crohn's disease. *Inflamm Bowel Dis* 2002; **8**: 10–15.

161. Borgaonkar MR, MacIntosh DG, Fardy JM. A meta-analysis of antimicrobacterial therapy for Crohn's disease. *Am J Gastroenterol* 2000; **95**: 725–9.

162. Colombel JF, Ferrari N, Debuysere H et al. Genotypic analysis of thiopurine *S*-methyltransferase in patients with Crohn's disease and severe myelosuppression during azathioprine therapy. *Gastroenterology* 2000; **118**: 1025–30.

163. Nielsen OH, Vainer B, Rask-Madsen J. Review article: the treatment of inflammatory bowel disease with 6-mercaptopurine or azathioprine. *Aliment Pharmacol Ther* 2001; **15**: 1699–708.

164. Lennard L. TPMT in the treatment of Crohn's disease with azathioprine. *Gut* 2002; **51**: 143–6.

165. Danielsson DE, Persson S. Antibacterial activity of azathioprine (Imuran) against anaerobic intestinal bacteria: implications in Crohn's disease. *Curr Chemother* 1978; **8**: 295–8.

166. Sandborn WJ, Tremaine WJ, Wolf DC et al. Lack of effect of intravenous administration on time to respond to azathioprine for steroid-treated Crohn's disease. *Gastroenterology* 1999; **117**: 527–35.

167. Candy S, Wright J, Gerber M et al. A controlled double blind study of azathioprine in the management of Crohn's disease. *Gut* 1995; **37**: 674–8.

168. Pearson DC, May GR, Fick GH et al. Azathioprine and 6-mercaptopurine in Crohn's disease: a meta-analysis. *Ann Intern Med* 1995; **122**: 132–42.

169. Pearson DC, May GR, Fick G et al. Azathioprine for maintaining remission of Crohn's disease. In: *The Cochrane Library*. Oxford: The Cochrane Collaboration, Update Software, 1999; issue 2.

170. Lemann M, Bouhnik Y, Colombel J-F et al. Randomized, double-blind, placebo-controlled, multicentre azathioprine withdrawal trial in Crohn's disease. *Gastroenterology* 2002; **122**: A34 (abstract).

171. McGovern DPB, Travis SPL, Duley J et al. Azathioprine intolerance in patients with IBD may be imidazole-related and is independent of TPMT activity. *Gastroenterology* 2002; **122**: 838–9.

172. Boulton-Jones JR, Pritchard K, Mahmoud AA. The use of 6-mercaptopurine in patients with inflammatory bowel disease after failure of azathioprine therapy. *Aliment Pharmacol Ther* 2000; **14**: 1561–5.

173. Bowen DG, Selby WS. Use of 6-mercaptopurine in patients with inflammatory bowel disease previously intolerant of azathioprine. *Dig Dis Sci* 2000; **45**: 1810–13.

174. Castiglione F, del Vecchio Blanco G, Rispo A et al. Hepatitis related to cytomegalovirus infection in two patients with Crohn's disease treated with azathioprine. *Dig Liver Dis* 2000; **32**: 626–9.

175. Kinlen LJ, Sheil AGR, Peto J et al. Collaborative United Kingdom–Australian study of cancer in patients treated with immunosuppressive drugs. *Br Med J* 1979; **ii**: 1461–6.

176. Dayharsh GA, Loftus EV, Sandborn WJ et al. *Epstein-Barr* virus positive lymphoma in patients with inflammatory bowel disease treated with azathioprine or 6-mercaptopurine. *Gastroenterology* 2002; **122**: 72–7.

177. Austin AS, Spiller RC. Inflammatory bowel disease, azathioprine and skin cancer: case report and literature review. *Eur J Gastroenterol Hepatol* 2001; **13**: 193–4.

178. Connell WR, Kamm MA, Dickson M et al. Long-term neoplasia risk after azathioprine treatment in inflammatory bowel disease. *Lancet* 1994; **343**: 1249–52.

179. Alstead EM, Ritchie JR, Lennard-Jones JE et al. Safety of azathioprine in pregnancy and inflammatory bowel disease. *Gastroenterology* 1990; **99**: 443–6.

180. Francella A, Dyan A, Bodian C et al. The safety of 6-mercaptopurine for child-bearing patients with inflammatory bowel disease: a retrospective cohort study. *Gastroenterology* 2003; **124**: 9–17.

181. Janssen NM, Genta MS. The effects of immunosuppressive and anti-inflammatory medications on fertility, pregnancy, and lactation. *Arch Int Med* 2000; **160**: 610–19.

182. Rajapakse R, Korelitz BI. Inflammatory bowel disease during pregnancy. *Curr Treat Opt Gastroenterol* 2001; **4**: 245–51.

183. Dejaco C, Mittermaier C, Reinisch W et al. Azathioprine treatment and male fertility in inflammatory bowel disease. *Gastroenterology* 2001; **121**: 1048–53.

184. Connell WR, Kamm MA, Ritchie JK et al. Bone marrow toxicity caused by azathioprine in inflammatory bowel disease. *Gut* 1993; **34**: 1081–5.

185. Cuffari C, Hunt S, Bayless T. Utilisation of erythrocyte 6-thioguanine metabolite levels to optimise azathioprine therapy in patients with inflammatory bowel disease. *Gut* 2001; **48**: 642–6.

186. Campbell S, Ghosh S. Is neutropenia required for effective maintenance of remission during azathioprine therapy in inflammatory bowel disease? *Eur J Gastroenterol Hepatol* 2001; **13**: 1073–6.

187. Jobson B, Garza A, Sninsky CA. Red cell mean corpuscular volume (MCV) correlates with 6-thioguanine nucleotide (6TG) levels during azathioprine or 6-MP therapy for Crohn's disease. *Gastroenterology* 2001; **120**(Suppl 1): 18.

188. Dubinsky MC, Hassard PV, Seidman EG et al. An open-label pilot study using thioguanine as a therapeutic alternative in Crohn's disease patients resistant to 6-mercaptopurine therapy. *Inflamm Bowel Dis* 2001; **7**: 181–9.

189. Korelitz B, Hanauer S, Rutgeerts P et al. Post-operative prophylaxis with 6-MP, 5-ASA or placebo in Crohn's disease: a two year multi-centre trial. *Gastroenterology* 1998; **114**: G4141 (abstract).

190. Cuillerier E, Lemann M, Bouhnik Y et al. Azathioprine for prevention of postoperative recurrence in Crohn's disease: a retrospective study. *Eur J Gastroenterol Hepatol* 2001; **13**: 1291–6.

191. Baert F, Noman M, Vermeire S et al. Influence of immunogenicity on the long-term efficacy of infliximab in Crohn's disease. *N Engl J Med* 2003; **348**: 601–8.

192. Zins BJ, Sandborn WJ, McKinney JA et al. A dose-ranging study of azathioprine pharmacokinetics after single-dose administration of a delayed-release oral formulation. *J Clin Pharmacol* 1997; **37**: 38–46.

193. Egan LJ, Sandborn WJ. Methotrexate for inflammatory bowel disease: pharmacology and preliminary results. *Mayo Clin Proc* 1996; **71**: 69–80.

194. Rampton DS. Methotrexate in Crohn's disease. *Gut* 2001; **48**: 790–1.

195. Feagan BG, Rochon J, Fedorak RN et al. Methotrexate for the treatment of Crohn's disease. The North American Crohn's Study Group Investigators. *N Engl J Med* 1995; **332**: 292–7.

196. Oren R, Moshkowitz M, Odes S et al. Methotrexate in chronic active Crohn's disease: a double-blind, randomised, Israeli multicentre trial. *Am J Gastroenterol* 1997; **92**: 2203–9.

197. Arora S, Katkov W, Cooley J et al. Methotrexate in Crohn's disease: results of a randomised, double-blind, placebo-controlled trial. *Hepatogastroenterology* 1999; **46**: 1724–9.

198. Egan LS, Sandborn WJ, Tremaine WJ et al. A randomised dose–response and pharmacokinetic study of methotrexate for refractory inflammatory Crohn's disease and ulcerative colitis. *Aliment Pharmacol Ther* 1999; **13**: 1597–604.

199. Feagan BG, Fedorak RN, Irvine EJ et al. A comparison of methotrexate with placebo for the maintenance of remission in Crohn's disease. North American Crohn's Study Group Investigators. *N Engl J Med* 2000; **342**: 1664–6.

200. Morgan SL, Baggott JE, Vaughn WH et al. Supplementation with folic acid during methotrexate therapy for rheumatoid arthritis. A double-blind, placebo-controlled trial. *Ann Intern Med* 1994; **121**: 833–41.

201. Kremer JM, Alarcon GS, Lightfoot RW et al. Methotrexate for rheumatoid arthritis: suggested guidelines for monitoring liver toxicity: American College of Rheumatology. *Arthritis Rheum* 1994; **37**: 316–28.

202. Te HS, Schiano TD, Kuan SF et al. Hepatic effects of long-term methotrexate use in the treatment of inflammatory bowel disease. *Am J Gastroenterol* 2000; **95**: 3150–6.

203. Lipsky JJ. Mycophenolate mofetil. *Lancet* 1996; **348**: 1357–9.

204. Neurath MF, Wanitschke R, Peters M et al. Randomised trial of mycophenolate mofetil versus azathioprine for treatment of chronic active Crohn's disease. *Gut* 1999; **44**: 625–8.

205. Fickert P, Hinterleitner TA, Wenzl HH et al. Mycophenolate mofetil in patients with Crohn's disease. *Am J Gastroenterol* 1998; **93**: 2529–32.

206. Lowry PW, Sandborn WJ, Lipsky JJ. Mycophenolate mofetil for Crohn's disease. *Lancet* 1999; **354**: 3–4.
207. Miehsler W, Reinisch W, Moser G et al. Is mycophenolate mofetil an effective alternative in azathioprine-intolerant patients with chronic active Crohn's disease? *Am J Gastroenterol* 2001; **96**: 782–7.
208. Fellermann K, Steffen M, Stein J et al. Mycophenolate mofetil: lack of efficacy in chronic active inflammatory bowel disease. *Aliment Pharmacol Ther* 2000; **14**: 171–6.
209. Hassard PV, Vasiliauskas EA, Kam LY et al. Efficacy of mycophenolate mofetil in patients failing 6-mercaptopurine or azathioprine therapy for Crohn's disease. *Inflamm Bowel Dis* 2000; **6**: 16–20.
210. Skelly MM, Logan RF, Jenkins D et al. Toxicity of mycophenolate mofetil in patients with inflammatory bowel disease. *Inflamm Bowel Dis* 2002; **8**: 93–7.
211. Lichtiger S, Present DH, Kornbluth A et al. Cyclosporine in severe ulcerative colitis refractory to steroid therapy. *N Engl J Med* 1994; **330**: 1841–5.
212. Brynskov J, Freund L, Rasmussen SN et al. A placebo-controlled, double-blind randomised trial of cyclosporin therapy in active Crohn's disease. *N Engl J Med* 1989; **321**: 845–50.
213. Brynskov J, Freund L, Rasmussen SN et al. Final report on a placebo-controlled, double-blind, randomised, multicentre trial of cyclosporin treatment in active Crohn's disease. *Scand J Gastroenterol* 1991; **26**: 689–95.
214. Feagan BG, McDonald JW, Rochon J et al. Low-dose cyclosporine for the treatment of Crohn's disease. The Canadian Crohn's Relapse Prevention Trial Investigators. *N Engl J Med* 1994; **330**: 1846–51.
215. Egan LS, Sandborn WJ, Tremaine WJ. Clinical outcome following treatment of refractory inflammatory and fistulizing Crohn's disease with intravenous cyclosporine. *Am J Gastroenterol* 1998; **93**: 442–8.
216. Korelitz BI. Inflammatory bowel disease and pregnancy. *Gastroenterol Clin North Am* 1998; **27**: 213–24.
217. Sandborn WJ. A critical review of cyclosporine therapy in inflammatory bowel disease. *Inflamm Bowel Dis* 1995; **1**: 48–63.
218. Langmead L, Rampton DS. Herbal treatment in gastrointestinal and liver disease – benefits and dangers. *Aliment Pharmacol Ther* 2001; **15**: 1239–52.
219. Sandborn WJ. Preliminary report on the use of oral tacrolimus (FK506) in the treatment of complicated proximal small bowel and fistulizing Crohn's disease. *Am J Gastroenterol* 1997; **92**: 876–9.
220. Sandborn WJ, Present DH, Isaccs KL et al. Tacrolimus (FK506) for the treatment of perianal and enterocutaneous fistulas in patients with Crohn's disease: a randomised, double-blind, placebo-controlled trial. *Gastroenterology* 2002; **122**: A136 (abstract).
221. Ierardi E, Principi M, Francavilla R et al. Oral tacrolimus long-term therapy in patients with Crohn's disease and steroid resistance. *Aliment Pharmacol Ther* 2001; **15**: 371–7.
222. Casson DH, Eltumi M, Tomlin S et al. Topical tacrolimus may be effective in the treatment of oral and perineal Crohn's disease. *Gut* 2000; **47**: 436–40.
223. Stallmach A, Wittig BM, Moser C et al. Safety and efficacy of intravenous pulse cyclophosphamide in acute steroid-refractory inflammatory bowel disease. *Gut* 2003; **52**: 377–82.
224. van Deventer SJ. Transmembrane TNF-alpha, induction of apoptosis, and the efficacy of TNF-targeting therapies in Crohn's disease. *Gastroenterology* 2001; **121**: 1242–6.
225. Baert FJ, D'Haens GR, Peeters M et al. Tumor necrosis factor alpha antibody (infliximab) therapy profoundly down-regulates the inflammation in Crohn's ileocolitis. *Gastroenterology* 1999; **116**: 22–8.

226. Feldmann M, Maini RN. Anti-TNF alpha therapy of rheumatoid arthritis: what have we learned? *Annu Rev Immunol* 2001; **19**: 163–96.
227. Targan SR, Hanauer SB, van Deventer SJH et al. A short-term study of chimeric monoclonal antibody cA2 to tumour necrosis alpha for Crohn's disease. *N Engl J Med* 1999; **337**: 1029–35.
228. Stack WA, Mann SD, Roy AJ et al. Randomised controlled trial of CDP571 antibody to tumour necrosis factor-alpha in Crohn's disease. *Lancet* 1997; **349**: 521–4.
229. Sandborn WJ, Feagan BG, Hanauer SB et al. An engineered human antibody to TNF (CDP571) for active Crohn's disease: a randomized double-blind placebo-controlled trial. *Gastroenterology* 2001; **120**: 1330–8.
230. Rutgeerts P, D'Haens G, Targan S et al. Efficacy and safety of retreatment with anti-tumor necrosis factor antibody (infliximab) to maintain remission in Crohn's disease. *Gastroenterology* 1999; **117**: 761–9.
231. Hanauer SB, Feagan BG, Lichtenstein GR et al. Maintenance infliximab for Crohn's disease: the ACCENT 1 randomised trial. *Lancet* 2002; **359**: 1541–9.
232. NICE. *Guidance on the Use of Infliximab for Crohn's Disease*, Technology Appraisal Guidance. No. 40. London: National Institute for Clinical Excellence, 2002.
233. Sands BE, van Deventer S, Bernstein C et al. Longterm treatment of fistulizing Crohn's disease: response to infliximab in the ACCENT II trial through 54 weeks. *Gastroenterology* 2002; **122**: A136.
234. Van Assche G, Vanbeckevoort D, Bielen D et al. Magnetic resonance imaging of the effects of infliximab in perianal fistulizing Crohn's disease. *Am J Gastroenterol* 2003; **98**: 332–9.
235. Arseneau KO, Cohn SM, Cominelli F et al. Cost-utility of initial medical management for Crohn's disease. *Gastroenterology* 2001; **120**: 1640–56.
236. Maini RN, Breedveld FC, Kalden JR et al. Therapeutic efficacy of multiple intravenous infusions of anti-tumor necrosis factor alpha monoclonal antibody combined with low-dose weekly methotrexate in rheumatoid arthritis. *Arthritis Rheum* 1998; **41**: 1552–63.
237. Vermeire S, Louis E, Carbonez A et al. Logistic regression of clinical parameters influencing response to infliximab. *Gastroenterology* 2001; **120**(Suppl 1): 3149 (abstract).
238. Parsi MA, Achkar JP, Richardson S et al. Predictors of response to infliximab in patients with Crohn's disease. *Gastroenterology* 2002; **123**: 707–13.
239. Bickston SJ, Lichtenstein GR, Arseneau KO et al. The relationship between infliximab treatment and lymphoma in Crohn's disease. *Gastroenterology* 1999; **117**: 1433–7.
240. Feagan BG, Sandborn WJ, Baker JP et al. A randomized, double-blind, placebo-controlled, multi-center trial of the engineered human antibody to TNF (CDP571) for steroid sparing and maintenance of remission in patients with steroid-dependent Crohn's disease. *Gastroenterology* 2000; **118**(Suppl 4): 3599 (abstract).
241. Sandborn WJ, Hanauer SB, Katz S et al. Etanercept for active Crohn's disease: a randomized, double-blind, placebo-controlled trial. *Gastroenterology* 2001; **121**: 1088–94.
242. Keane J, Gershon S, Wise RP et al. Tuberculosis associated with infliximab, a tumor necrosis factor alpha-neutralizing agent. *N Engl J Med* 2001; **345**: 1098–104.
243. de Rosa FG, Bonora S, Di Perri G. Tuberculosis and treatment with infliximab. *N Engl J Med* 2002; **346**: 623–6.
244. Anonymous. Heart failure on infliximab. *Prescrire Int* 2002; **11**: 86–7.
245. Marotte H, Charrin JE, Miossec P. Infliximab-induced aseptic meningitis. *Lancet* 2001; **358**: 1784.

246. van Oosten BW, Barkhof F, Truyen L et al. Increased MRI activity and immune activation in two multiple sclerosis patients treated with the monoclonal anti-tumor necrosis factor antibody cA2. *Neurology* 1996; **47**: 1531–4.

247. Prajapati DN, Satian K, Kim JP et al. Symptomatic luminal stricture underlies infliximab non-response in Crohn's disease. *Gastroenterology* 2002; **122**: A152 (abstract).

248. Katz JA, Lichtenstein GR, Keenan GF et al. Outcome of pregnancy in women receiving Remicade (infliximab) for the treatment of Crohn's disease or rheumatoid arthritis. *Gastroenterology* 2001; **120**: A69 (abstract).

249. Kugathasan S, Levy MB, Saeian K et al. Infliximab retreatment in adults and children with Crohn's disease: risk factors for the development of delayed severe systemic reaction. *Am J Gastroenterol* 2002; **97**: 1408–14.

250. Cohen RD, Tsang JF, Hanauer SB. Infliximab in Crohn's disease: first anniversary clinical experience. *Am J Gastroenterol* 2000; **95**: 3469–77.

251. Sandborn WJ, Hanauer SB. Infliximab in the treatment of Crohn's disease: a users guide for clinicians. *Am J Gastroenterol* 2002; **97**: 2962–72.

252. Alsahli M, Yoon-Tae J, Peppercorn MA et al. A randomized, double-blind, placebo-controlled trial of intravenous hydrocortisone in reducing human antichimeric antibody following infliximab infusion. *Gastroenterology* 2002; **122**: A156 (abstract).

253. Markham A, Lamb HM. Infliximab: a review of its use in the management of rheumatoid arthritis. *Drugs* 2000; **59**: 1341–59.

254. Mow WS, Abreu MT, Papadakis KA et al. High incidence of anergy limits the usefulness of PPD screening for tuberculosis prior to Remicade in inflammatory bowel disease. *Gastroenterology* 2002; **122**: A156 (abstract).

255. Aberra FN, McGregor J, Brennan PR et al. Is a PPD skin test result sufficient in determining risk of reactivation of latent TB infection in IBD patients that are candidates for infliximab therapy? *Gastroenterology* 2002; **122**: A855 (abstract).

256. Caprilli R, Viscido A, Guagnozzi D. Review article: biological agents in the treatment of Crohn's disease. *Aliment Pharmacol Ther* 2002; **16**: 1579–90.

257. de Silva AP, Vermeire S, Ahmad T et al. Pharmacogenetics of infliximab in Crohn's disease: the 5q31/IBD5 risk haplotype predicts response. *Gastroenterology* 2002; **122**: A395 (abstract).

258. Bauditz J, Wedel S, Lochs H. Thalidomide reduces tumour necrosis factor alpha and interleukin 12 production in patients with chronic active Crohn's disease. *Gut* 2002; **50**: 196–200.

259. Vasiliauskas EA, Kam LY, Abreu-Martin MT et al. An open-label pilot study of low-dose thalidomide in chronically active, steroid-dependent Crohn's disease. *Gastroenterology* 1999; **117**: 1278–87.

260. Ginsburg PM, Hanan I, Ehrenpreis ED. Treatment of severe esophageal Crohn's disease with thalidomide. *Am J Gastroenterol* 2001; **96**: 1305–6.

261. Rutgeerts P, Lemmens L, van Assche G et al. Treatment of active Crohn's disease with Onercept (recombinant human soluble p55 tumour necrosis factor receptor): results of a randomized, open-label, pilot study. *Aliment Pharmacol Ther* 2003; **17**: 185–92.

262. Hommes DW, van den Blink B, Plasse T et al. Inhibition of stress-activated MAP-kinases induces clinical improvement in moderate to severe Crohn's disease. *Gastroenterology* 2002; **122**: 7–14.

263. Summers RW, Urban J, Elliott D et al. Th2 conditioning by *Trichuris suis* appears safe and effective in modifying the mucosal immune response in inflammatory bowel disease. *Gastroenterology* 1999; **116**: A828 (abstract).

264. Steidler L, Hans W, Schotte L et al. Treatment of murine colitis by *Lactobacillus lactis* secreting interleukin-10. *Science* 2000; **289**: 1352–5.

265. Walters CF, Heineman E, Thunnissen FB et al. Effect of dietary inulin supplementation in inflammation of pouch mucosa in patients with ileopouch–anal anastomosis. *Dis Colon Rectum* 2002; **45**: 621–7.
266. Kruis W, Schutz E, Fric P et al. Double-blind comparison of an oral *Escherichia coli* preparation and mesalazine in maintaining remission in ulcerative colitis. *Aliment Pharmacol Ther* 1997; **11**: 853–8.
267. Rembacken BJ, Snelling AM, Hawkey PM et al. Non-pathogenic *Escherichia coli* versus mesalazine for the treatment of ulcerative colitis: a randomised trial. *Lancet* 1999; **354**: 635–9.
268. Gionchetti P, Rizzello F, Venturi A et al. Oral bacteriotherapy as maintenance treatment in patients with chronic pouchitis: a double-blind, placebo-controlled trial. *Gastroenterology* 2000; **119**: 305–9.
269. Guslandi M, Mezzi G, Sorghi M et al. *Saccharomyces boulardii* in maintenance treatment of Crohn's disease. *Dig Dis Sci* 2000; **45**: 1462–4.
270. Rautio M, Jousimies-Somer H, Kauma H et al. Liver abscess due to a *Lactobacillus rhamnosus* strain indistinguishable from *L. rhamnosus* strain GG. *Clin Infect Dis* 1999; **28**: 1159–60.
271. Vernia P, Marcheggiano A, Caprilli R et al. Short-chain fatty acid topical treatment in distal ulcerative colitis. *Aliment Pharmacol Ther* 1995; **9**: 309–13.
272. Breuer RI, Soergel KH, Lashner BA et al. Short chain fatty acid rectal irrigation for left-sided ulcerative colitis: a randomised, placebo controlled trial. *Gut* 1997; **40**: 485–91.
273. Slonim AE, Bulone L, Damore MB et al. A preliminary study of growth hormone therapy for Crohn's disease. *N Engl J Med* 2000; **342**: 1633–7.
274. Kosaka T, Sawada K, Ohnishi K et al. Effect of leukocytopheresis therapy using a leukocyte removal filter in Crohn's disease. *Intern Med* 1999; **38**: 102–111.
275. Lopez-Cubero SO, Sullivan KM, McDonald GB. Course of Crohn's disease after allogenic bone marrow transplantation. *Gastroenterology* 1998; **114**: 433–40.
276. Craig RM, Oyama Y, Traynor AE et al. Autologous hematopoietic stem cell transplantation for refractory Crohn's disease. *Gastroenterology* 2002; **122**: A432 (abstract).
277. Stronkhorst A, Radema S, Yong SL et al. CD4 antibody treatment in patients with active Crohn's disease: a phase 1 dose finding study. *Gut* 1997; **40**: 320–7.
278. James SP. Remission of Crohn's disease after human immunodeficiency virus infection. *Gastroenterology* 1988; **95**: 1667–9.
279. Sharpstone DR, Duggal A, Gazzard BG. Inflammatory bowel disease in individuals seropositive for the human immunodeficiency virus. *Eur J Gastroenterol Hepatol* 1996; **8**: 575–8.
280. Schreiber S, Nikolaus S, Malchow H et al. Absence of efficacy of subcutaneous ICAM-1 treatment of chronic active Crohn's disease. *Gastroenterology* 2001; **120**: 1339–46.
281. Yacyshyn BR, Chey WY, Goff J et al. Double blind, placebo-controlled trial of the remission and steroid sparing properties of an ICAM-1 antisense oligodeoxynucleotide, alicaforsen (ISIS 2302), in active steroid dependent Crohn's disease. *Gut* 2002; **51**: 30–6.
282. Gordon FH, Lai CW, Hamilton MI et al. A randomized placebo-controlled trial of a humanized monoclonal antibody to alpha4 integrin in active Crohn's disease. *Gastroenterology* 2001; **121**: 268–74.
283. Ghosh S, Goldin E, Malchow HA et al. A randomised, double-blind, placebo-controlled, pan-European study of a recombinant humanised antibody to α4 integrin (Antegren™) in moderate to severely active Crohn's disease. *Gastroenterology* 2001; **120**(Suppl 1): 682 (abstract).
284. Vangham D, Drumm B. Treatment of fistulas with G-CSF in a patient with Crohn's disease. *N Engl J Med* 1999; **340**: 239–40.

285. Bourreille A, Doubremelle M, de la Blétière DR et al. RDP 1258, a novel immunomodulatory peptide, decreases tumor necrosis factor in Crohn's disease and suppresses inflammation in experimental colitis. *Gastroenterology* 2001; **120**(Suppl 1): 3703 (abstract).

286. Strober W, Ludviksson BR, Fuss IJ. The pathogenesis of mucosal inflammation in murine models of inflammatory bowel disease and Crohn's disease. *Ann Intern Med* 1998; **128**: 848–56.

287. Lindsay JO, Hodgson HJ. Review article: the immunoregulatory cytokine interleukin-10 – a therapy for Crohn's disease? *Aliment Pharmacol Ther* 2001; **15**: 1709–16.

288. van Deventer SJ, Elson CO, Fedorak RN. Multiple doses of intravenous interleukin-10 in steroid-refractory Crohn's disease. Crohn's Disease Study Group. *Gastroenterology* 1997; **113**: 383–9.

289. Fedorak RN, Gangl A, Elson CO et al. Recombinant human interleukin-10 in the treatment of patients with mild to moderately active Crohn's disease. The interleukin-10 Inflammatory Bowel Disease Cooperative Study Group. *Gastroenterology* 2000; **119**: 1473–82.

290. Schreiber S, Fedorak RN, Nielsen OH et al. Safety and efficacy of recombinant human interleukin 10 in chronic active Crohn's disease. Crohn's disease IL-10 Cooperative Study Group. *Gastroenterology* 2000; **119**: 1461–72.

291. Colombel JF, Rutgeerts P, Malchow H et al. Interleukin 10 (Tenovil) in the prevention of postoperative recurrence of Crohn's disease. *Gut* 2001; **49**: 42–6.

292. Sands BE, Bank S, Sninsky CA et al. Preliminary evaluation of safety and activity of recombinant human interleukin 11 in patients with active Crohn's disease. *Gastroenterology* 1999; **117**: 58–64.

293. Sands BE, Winston BD, Salzberg B et al. Randomized, controlled trial of recombinant human interleukin-11 in patients with active Crohn's disease. *Aliment Pharmacol Ther* 2002; **16**: 399–406.

294. Reuter BK, Asfaha S, Buret A et al. Exacerbation of inflammation-associated colonic injury in rat through inhibition of cyclooxygenase-2. *J Clin Invest* 1996; **98**: 2076–85.

295. Hawkey CJ, Dube LM, Rountree LV et al. A trial of zileuton versus mesalazine or placebo in the maintenance of remission of ulcerative colitis. The European Zileuton Study Group for Ulcerative Colitis. *Gastroenterology* 1997; **112**: 718–24.

296. Carty E, Rampton DS, Schneider H et al. Lack of efficacy of ridogrel, a thromboxane synthase inhibitor, in a placebo-controlled, double-blind, multi-centre clinical trial in active Crohn's disease. *Aliment Pharmacol Ther* 2001; **15**: 1323–9.

297. Emerit J, Pelletier S, Tosoni-Verlignue D et al. Phase II trial of copper zinc superoxide dismutase (CuZnSOD) in treatment of Crohn's disease. *Free Radic Biol Med* 1989; **7**: 145–9.

298. Hawkes ND, Richardson C, Ch'Ng CL et al. Enteric-release glyceryl trinitrate in active Crohn's disease: a randomized, double-blind, placebo-controlled trial. *Aliment Pharmacol Ther* 2001; **15**: 1867–73.

299. Lorenz-Meyer H, Bauer P, Nicolay C et al. Omega-3 fatty acids and low carbohydrate diet for maintenance of remission in Crohn's disease. A randomized controlled multicenter trial. Study Group Members (German Crohn's Disease Study Group). *Scand J Gastroenterol* 1996; **31**: 778–85.

300. Belluzzi A, Brignola C, Campieri M et al. Effect of an enteric-coated fish-oil preparation on relapses in Crohn's disease. *N Engl J Med* 1996; **334**: 1557–60.

301. Neurath MF, Petterson S, Meyer zum Buschenfelde KH et al. Local administration of antisense phosphorothioate oligonucleotides to the p65 subunit of NF-kappa B abrogates established experimental colitis in mice. *Nature Med* 1996; **2**: 998–1004.

302. Löfberg R, Neurath M, Ost A et al. Topical NFκB p65 antisense oligonucleotides in patients with active distal colonic IBD. A randomized, controlled pilot trial. *Gastroenterology* 2002; **122**: A102 (abstract).

303. Berger J, Moller DE. The mechanisms of action of PPARs. *Annu Rev Med* 2002; **53**: 409–35.

304. Bjorck S, Dahlstrom A, Ahlman H. Treatment of distal ulcerative colitis with lidocaine. *Can J Gastroenterol* 1993; **7**: 179–81.

305. Papa A, Danese S, Gasbarrini A et al. Review article: potential therapeutic applications and mechanisms of action of heparin in inflammatory bowel disease. *Aliment Pharmacol Ther* 2000; **14**: 1403–9.

306. Day R, Forbes A. Heparin, cell adhesion, and pathogenesis of inflammatory bowel disease. *Lancet* 1999; **354**: 62–5.

307. Panes J, Esteve M, Cabre E et al. Comparison of heparin and steroids in the treatment of moderate and severe ulcerative colitis. *Gastroenterology* 2000; **119**: 903–8.

308. Ang YS, Mahmud N, White B et al. Randomized comparison of unfractionated heparin with corticsteroids in severe active inflammatory bowel disease. *Aliment Pharmacol Ther* 2000; **14**: 1015–22.

309. Folwaczny C, Wiebecke B, Loeschke K. Unfractionated heparin in the therapy of patients with highly active inflammatory bowel disease. *Am J Gastroenterol* 1999; **94**: 1551–5.

310. Jalan KN, Sircus W, Card WI et al. An experience of UC. I. Toxic dilatation in 55 cases. *Gastroenterology* 1969; **57**: 68–82.

311. Hofmann AF, Poley JR. Role of bile acid malabsorption in the pathogenesis of diarrhoea and steatorrhoea in patients with ileal resection. I. Response to cholestyramine or replacement of dietary long chain triglycerides by medium chain triglycerides. *Gastroenterology* 1972; **62**: 918–34.

312. Rampton DS. Medical management: how can efficacy and safety be maximised? In: Rampton DS, ed. *Inflammatory Bowel Disease, Clinical Diagnosis and Management*. London: Martin Dunitz Ltd, 2000, 143–84.

313. Dubinsky MC, Lamothe S, Yang HY et al. Pharmacogenomics and metabolite measurement for 6-mercaptopurine therapy in inflammatory bowel disease. *Gastroenterology* 2000; **118**: 705–13.

314. Mekhijan HS, Sweitz DM, Watts HD et al. National cooperative Crohn's disease study: factors determining recurrence of Crohn's disease after surgery. *Gastroenterology* 1979; **77**: 907–13.

315. Ekelund GR, Lindhagen T. Controversies in the surgical management of Crohn's disease. *Perspect Colon Rectal Surg* 1989; **2**: 1–14.

316. Lipson AB, Savage MO, Davies PS et al. Acceleration of linear growth following intestinal resection for Crohn's disease. *Eur J Paediatrics* 1990; **149**: 687.

317. Rombeau JL, Barot LR, Williamson CE et al. Preoperative total parenteral nutrition and surgical outcome in patients with inflammatory bowel disease. *Am J Surg* 1982; **143**: 139–43.

318. Ellis LM, Copeland EM, Souba WW. Perioperative nutritional support. *Surg Clin North Am* 1991; **71**: 493–507.

319. Delaney CP, Fazio VW. Crohn's disease of the small bowel. *Surg Clin North Am* 2001; **81**: 137–58.

320. Bergman L, Krause U. Crohn's disease: a long-term study of the clinical course in 186 patients. *Scand J Gastroenterol* 1977; **12**: 937–44.

321. Fazio VW, Marchetti F, Church JM et al. Effect of resection margins on the recurrence of Crohn's disease in the small bowel: a randomised controlled trial. *Ann Surg* 1996; **224**: 563–73.

322. Hashemi M, Novell JR, Lewis AA. Side-to-side stapled anastomosis may delay recurrence in Crohn's disease. *Dis Colon Rectum* 1998; **41**: 1293–6.

323. Munoz-Juarez M, Yamamoto T, Wolff BG et al. Wide-lumen stapled anastomosis vs conventional end-to-end anastomosis in the treatment of Crohn's disease. *Dis Colon Rectum* 2001; **44**: 20–5.

324. Rutgeerts P, Geboes K, Vantrappen G et al. Natural history of recurrent Crohn's disease at the ileocolonic anastomosis after curative surgery. *Gut* 1984; **25**: 665–72.

325. McLeod RS, Wolff BG, Steinhart AH et al. Risk and significance of endoscopic/radiological evidence of recurrent Crohn's disease. *Gastroenterology* 1997; **113**: 1823–7.

326. Heimann TM, Greenstein AJ, Lewis B et al. Prediction of early symptomatic recurrence after intestinal recurrence in Crohn's disease. *Ann Surg* 1993; **218**: 294–8.

327. Greenstein AJ, Sachar DB, Pasternack BS et al. Reoperation and recurrence in Crohn's colitis and ileocolitis. *N Engl J Med* 1975; **293**: 685–90.

328. Lee ECG, Papaioannou N. Minimal surgery for chronic obstruction in patients with extensive or universal Crohn's disease. *Ann R Coll Surg Engl* 1982; **64**: 229–33.

329. Stebbing JF, Jewell DP, Kettlewell MGW et al. Long-term results of recurrence and reoperation after strictureplasty for obstructive Crohn's disease. *Br J Surg* 1995; **82**: 1471–4.

330. Ozuner G, Fazio VW, Lavery IC et al. How safe is strictureplasty in the management of Crohn's disease? *Am J Surg* 1996; **171**: 57–61.

331. Couckuyt H, Gevers AM, Coremans G et al. Efficacy and safety of hydrostatic balloon dilatation of ileocolonic Crohn's disease strictures: a prospective longterm analysis. *Gut* 1995; **36**: 577–80.

332. Ramboer C, Verhamme M, Dhondt E et al. Endoscopic treatment of stenosis in recurrence Crohn's disease with balloon dilatation combined with local corticosteroid injection. *Gastrointest Endosc* 1995; **42**: 252–5.

333. Lavy A. Triamcinolone improves outcome in Crohn's disease strictures. *Dis Colon Rectum* 1997; **40**: 184–6.

334. Michelassi F, Stella M, Balestracci T et al. Incidence, diagnosis and treatment of enteric and colorectal fistulae in patients with Crohn's disease. *Ann Surg* 1993; **218**: 660–6.

335. Matsui T, Hatakeyama S, Ikeda K et al. Long-term outcome of endoscopic balloon dilation in obstructive gastroduodenal Crohn's disease. *Endoscopy* 1997; **29**: 640–5.

336. Yamamoto T, Bain IM, Connolly AB et al. Gastroduodenal fistulas in Crohn's disease: clinical features and management. *Dis Colon Rectum* 1998; **41**: 1287–92.

337. Longo WE, Oakley JR, Lavery IC et al. Outcome of ileorectal anastomosis for Crohn's colitis. *Dis Colon Rectum* 1992; **35**: 1066–71.

338. Allan A, Andrews H, Hilton C et al. Segmental colonic resection is an appropriate operation for short skip lesions due to Crohn's disease of the colon. *World J Surg* 1989; **13**: 611–16.

339. Ambrose NS, Keighley MRB, Alexander-Williams J et al. Clinical impact of colectomy and ileorectal anastomosis in the management of Crohn's disease. *Gut* 1984; **25**: 223–7.

340. Fazio VW, Wu JS. Surgical therapy for Crohn's disease of the colon and rectum. *Surg Clin North Am* 1997; **77**: 197–210.

341. Cooper JC, Jones D, Williams NS. Outcome of colectomy and ileorectal anastomosis in Crohn's disease. *Ann R Coll Surg Engl* 1986; **68**: 279–82.

342. Chevalier JM, Jones DJ, Ratelle R et al. Colectomy and ileorectal anastomosis in patients with Crohn's disease. *Br J Surg* 1994; **81**: 1379–81.

343. Tjandra JJ, Fazio VW. Surgery of Crohn's colitis. *Int Surg* 1992; **77**: 9–14.

344. Sagar PM, Dozois RR, Wolff BG. Long-term results of ileal pouch–anal anastomosis in patients with Crohn's disease. *Br J Surg* 1995; **82**: 1629–33.
345. Winslet MC, Andrews H, Allan RH et al. Faecal diversion in the management of Crohn's disease of the colon. *Dis Colon Rectum* 1993; **36**: 757–62.
346. Guillem JG, Robert PL, Murray JJ et al. Factors predictive of persistent or recurrent Crohn's disease in excluded rectal segments. *Dis Colon Rectum* 1992; **35**: 768–72.
347. Steinberg DM, Allan RN, Thompson H et al. Excisional surgery with ileostomy for Crohn's colitis with particular reference to factors affecting recurrence. *Gut* 1974; **15**: 845–51.
348. Scammel BE, Andrews H, Allan RN et al. Results of proctocolectomy for Crohn's disease. *Br J Surg* 1987; **74**: 150–2.
349. Solomon MJ. Fistulae and abscesses in symptomatic perianal Crohn's. *Int J Colorect Dis* 1996; **11**: 222–6.
350. Kodner IJ. Perianal Crohn's disease. In: Allan RN, Rhodes JM, Hanauer SB et al, eds. *Inflammatory Bowel Diseases*, 3rd edition. New York: Churchill Livingstone, 1997, 863.
351. Williams DR, Collier JA, Corman ML et al. Anal complications of Crohn's disease. *Dis Colon Rectum* 1981; **24**: 22–4.
352. Keighley MRB, Allan RN. Current status and influence of operation on perianal Crohn's disease. *Int J Colorect Dis* 1986; **1**: 104–7.
353. Makowiec F, Jehle EC, Becker H et al. Perianal abscess in Crohn's disease. *Dis Colon Rectum* 1997; **40**: 443–50.
354. Buchmann P, Keighley MR, Allan RN et al. Natural history of perianal Crohn's disease. Ten year follow-up: a plea for conservatism. *Am J Surg* 1980; **140**: 642–4.
355. Fleshner P, Schoetz D, Roberts P et al. Anal fissure in Crohn's disease. A plea for aggressive management. *Dis Colon Rectum* 1995; **38**: 1137–43.
356. Sohn N, Korelitz, Weinstein MA. Anorectal Crohn's disease: definitive surgery for fistulas and recurrent abscesses. *Am J Surg* 1980; **139**: 394–7.
357. Williams JG, Rothernberger DA, Nemer FD et al. Fistula-in-ano in Crohn's disease: results of aggressive surgical treatment. *Dis Colon Rectum* 1991; **34**: 378–84.
358. Hellers G, Bergstrand O, Ewerth S et al. Occurrence and outcome after primary treatment of anal fistulae in Crohn's disease. *Gut* 1980; **21**: 525–7.
359. Williams JG, Wong WD, Rothenberger DA et al. Recurrence of Crohn's disease after resection. *Br J Surg* 1991; **78**: 10–19.
360. Linares L, Moreira LF, Andrews H et al. Natural history and treatment of anorectal strictures complicating Crohn's disease. *Br J Surg* 1988; **75**: 653–5.
361. Felt-Bersma R, Poen AC, Cuesta MA et al. Anal lesions and anorectal function in perianal Crohn's disease. *Gastroenterology* 1999; **116**: 714.
362. Wu JS, Birnbaum EH, Kodner IJ et al. Laparoscopic-assisted ileocolic resections in Crohn's patients: are abscesses, phlegmons, or recurrent disease contraindications? *Surgery* 1997; **122**: 682–8.
363. Bauer JJ, Harris MT, Grumbach NM et al. Laparoscopic-assisted intestinal resection: which patients are good candidates? *J Clin Gastroenterol* 1996; **23**: 44–6.
364. Ludwig KA, Milsom JW, Church JM et al. Preliminary experience with laparoscopic intestinal surgery for Crohn's disease. *Am J Surg* 1996; **171**: 52–6.
365. Reissmann P, Salky BA, Pfeifer J et al. Laparoscopic surgery in the management of inflammatory bowel disease. *Am J Surg* 1996; **171**: 47–51.
366. Milsom JW, Lavery IC, Bohm B et al. Laparoscopically-assisted ileocolectomy in Crohn's disease. *Surgical Endoscopy* 1993; **3**: 77–80.
367. Kreissler-Haag D, Hildebrandt U, Pistorius G et al. Laparoscopic surgery in Crohn's disease. *Surg Endosc* 1994; **8**: A1002 (abstract).

368. Ghanaiem A, Kiff R, O'Leary J et al. Laparoscopically assisted ileocolectomy for Crohn's disease. *Min Invas Therapy Allied Technol* 1996; 5: A491 (abstract).

369. Russell RI. Nutritional management: central importance in Crohn's disease but peripheral role in ulcerative colitis? In: Rampton DS, ed. *Inflammatory Bowel Disease, Clinical Diagnosis and Management.* London: Martin Dunitz Ltd, 2000, 185–207.

370. Dickinson RA, Ashton MG, Axon ATR et al. Controlled trial of intravenous hyperalimentation and total bowel rest as an adjunct to the routine therapy of acute colitis. *Gastroenterology* 1980; 79: 1199–204.

371. Elson CO, Layden TJ, Nemchausky BA et al. An evaluation of total parenteral nutrition in the management of inflammatory bowel disease. *Dig Dis Sci* 1980; 25: 42–8.

372. Muller JN, Keller HW, Erasmi H et al. Total parenteral nutrition as the sole therapy in Crohn's disease – a prospective study. *Br J Surg* 1983; 70: 40–3.

373. Schiloni E, Coronado E, Fruend H. Role of total parenteral nutrition in the treatment of Crohn's disease. *Am J Surg* 1989; 157: 180–5.

374. Seo M, Okada M, Yao T et al. The role of total parenteral nutrition in the management of patients with acute attacks of inflammatory bowel disease. *J Clin Gastroenterol* 1999; 29: 223–4.

375. Greenberg GR, Fleming CR, Jeejeebhoy KN et al. Controlled trial of bowel rest and nutritional support in the management of Crohn's disease. *Gut* 1988; 29: 1309–15.

376. Wright RA, Adler EC. Peripheral parenteral nutrition is no better than enteral nutrition in acute exacerbation of Crohn's disease – a prospective trial. *J Clin Gastroenterol* 1990; 12: 396–9.

377. Akobeng AK, Miller V, Stanton J et al. Double-blind randomized controlled trial of glutamine-enriched polymeric diet in the treatment of active Crohn's disease. *J Pediatr Gastroenterol Nutr* 2000; 30: 78–84.

378. Logan RFA, Gillon J, Ferrington C et al. Reduction of gastrointestinal protein loss by elemental diet in Crohn's disease of the small bowel. *Gut* 1981; 22: 383–7.

379. Teahon K, Smethurst P, Pearson N et al. The effect of elemental diet on intestinal permeability and inflammation in Crohn's disease. *Gastroenterology* 1991; 101: 84–9.

380. Gorard DA, Hunt JB, Payne-James JJ et al. Initial response and subsequent course of Crohn's disease treated with elemental diet or prednisolone. *Gut* 1993; 34: 1198–202.

381. Middleton SJ, Rucker JT, Kirby GA et al. Long-chain triglycerides reduce the efficacy of enteral feeds with active Crohn's disease. *Clin Nutr* 1995; 14: 229–36.

382. Leiper K, Woolner J, Mullan MM et al. A randomised controlled trial of high versus low long chain triglyceride whole protein feed in active Crohn's disease. *Gut* 2001; 49: 790–4.

383. Gassull MA, Fernandez-Benares F, Cabré E et al. Fat composition may be a clue to explain the primary therapeutic effect of enteral nutrition in Crohn's disease: results of a double blind randomised multicentre European trial. *Gut* 2002; 51: 164–8.

384. Walker-Smith JA, Phillips AD, Walford N et al. Intravenous epidermal growth factor/urogastrone increases small-intestinal cell proliferation in congenital microvillous atrophy. *Lancet* 1985; ii: 1239–40.

385. Fell JM, Paintin M, Arnaud-Battandier F et al. Mucosal healing and a fall in mucosal pro-inflammatory cytokine mRNA induced by a specific oral polymeric diet in paediatric Crohn's disease. *Aliment Pharmacol Ther* 2000; 14: 281–9.

386. Hilsden RJ, Hodgins D, Czechowsky D et al. Attitudes toward smoking and smoking behaviours of patients with Crohn's disease. *Am J Gastroenterol* 2001; 96: 1849–53.

387. Zollman C, Vickers A. ABC of complementary medicine. Users and practitioners of complementary medicine. *Br Med J* 1999; **319**: 836–8.
388. Rawsthorne P, Shanahan F, Cronin NC et al. An international survey of the use and attitudes regarding alternative medicine by patients with inflammatory bowel disease. *Am J Gastroenterol* 1999; **94**: 1298–303.
389. Hilsden RJ, Scott CM, Verhoef MJ. Complementary medicine use by patients with inflammatory bowel disease. *Am J Gastroenterol* 1998; **93**: 697–701.
390. Heuschkel R, Afzal N, Wuerth A et al. Complementary medicine use in children and young adults with inflammatory bowel disease. *Am J Gastroenterol* 2002; **97**: 382–8.
391. Langmead L, Chitnis M, Rampton DS. Use of complementary therapies by patients with inflammatory bowel disease indicates psychosocial distress. *Inflamm Bowel Dis* 2002; **8**: 174–9.
392. Mason S, Tovey P, Long AF. Evaluating complementary medicine: methodological challenges of randomised control trials. *Br Med J* 2002; **325**: 832–4.
393. Casellas F, Lopez-Vivancos J, Badia X et al. Influence of inflammatory bowel disease on different dimensions of quality of life. *Eur J Gastroenterol Hepatol* 2001; **13**: 567–72.
394. Kurina LM, Goldacre MJ, Yeates D et al. Depression and anxiety in patients with inflammatory bowel disease. *J Epidemiol Community Health* 2001; **55**: 716–20.
395. Anonymous. Risks of and prophylaxis for venous thromboembolism in hospital patients. Thromboembolic Risk Factors (THRIFT) Consensus Group. *Br Med J* 1992; **305**: 567–74.
396. McInerney GT, Sauer WG, Baggenstossa H et al. Fulminating ulcerative colitis with marked colonic dilatation: a clinicopathologic study. *Gastroenterology* 1962; **42**: 244–57.
397. Prantera C, Berto E, Scribano ML et al. Use of antibiotics in the treatment of active Crohn's disease: experience with metronidazole and ciprofloxacin. *Ital J Gastroenterol Hepatol* 1998; **30**: 593–8.
398. Modigliani R, Colombel JF, Dupas JL et al. Mesalamine in Crohn's disease with steroid-induced remission: effect on steroid withdrawal and remission maintenance. Groupe d'Etude Therapeutique des Affections Inflammatoires Digestives. *Gastroenterology* 1996; **110**: 688–93.
399. Stange EF, Modigliani R, Pena AS et al. European trial of cyclosporine in chronic active Crohn's disease: I. 12-month study. The European Study Group. *Gastroenterology* 1995; **109**: 774–82.
400. Bemelman WA, Ivenski M, van Hogezand RA et al. How effective is extensive nonsurgical treatment of patients with clinically active Crohn's disease of the terminal ileum in preventing surgery? *Dig Surg* 2001; **18**: 56–60.
401. Farthing MJG. Ileal Crohn's disease is best treated by surgery. *Gut* 2002; **50**: 13–14.
402. Windsor ACJ. Ileal Crohn's disease is best treated by surgery. *Gut* 2002; **50**: 11–12.
403. Pettit SH, Irving MH. The operative management of fistulous Crohn's disease. *Surg Gynecol Obstet* 1988; **167**: 223–8.
404. Jakobovitz J, Schuster MM. Metronidazole therapy for Crohn's disease and associated fistulae. *Am J Gastroenterol* 1984; **79**: 533–40.
405. Park JJ, Cintron JR, Orsay CP et al. Repair of chronic anorectal fistulae using commercial fibrin sealant. *Arch Surg* 2000; **135**: 166–9.
406. Korelitz BI, Adler DJ, Mendelsohn RA et al. Long-term experience with 6-mercaptopurine in the treatment of Crohn's disease. *Am J Gastroenterol* 1993; **88**: 1198–205.
407. Hanauer SB, Smith MB. Rapid closure of Crohn's disease fistulas with continuous intravenous cyclosporin A. *Am J Gastroenterol* 1993; **88**: 646–9.

408. Lowry PW, Weaver AL, Tremaine WJ et al. Combination therapy with oral tacrolimus (FK506) and azathioprine or 6-mercaptopurine for treatment-refractory Crohn's disease perianal fistulae. *Inflamm Bowel Dis* 1999; **5**: 239–45.

409. Valori RM, Cockel R. Omeprazole for duodenal ulceration in Crohn's disease. *Br Med J* 1990; **300**: 438–9.

410. Przemioslo RT, Mee AS. Omeprazole in possible esophageal Crohn's disease. *Dig Dis Sci* 1994; **39**: 1594–5.

411. Tyldesley WR. Oral Crohn's disease and related conditions. *Br J Oral Surg* 1979; **17**: 1–9.

412. Robertson LP, Hickling P. Treatment of recalcitrant orogenital ulceration of Behçet's syndrome with infliximab. *Rheumatology* 2001; **40**: 473–4.

413. Steinhart AH, Ewe K, Griffiths AM et al. Corticosteroids for maintaining remission of Crohn's disease. *Cochrane Database Syst Rev* 2001; CD000301.

414. Moum B, Ekbom A, Vatn MH et al. Clinical course during the 1st year after diagnosis in ulcerative colitis and Crohn's disease. *Scand J Gastroenterol* 1997; **32**: 1005–12.

415. Caprilli R, Andreoli A, Capurso L et al. Oral mesalazine (5-aminosalicylic acid; Asacol) for the prevention of post-operative recurrence of Crohn's disease. *Aliment Pharmacol Ther* 1994; **8**: 35–43.

416. Brignola C, Cottone M, Pera A et al. Mesalamine in the prevention of endoscopic recurrence after intestinal resection for Crohn's disease. Italian Cooperative Study Group. *Gastroenterology* 1995; **108**: 345–9.

417. McLeod RS, Wolff BG, Steinhart AH et al. Prophylactic mesalamine treatment decreases postoperative recurrence of Crohn's disease. *Gastroenterology* 1995; **109**: 404–13.

418. Sutherland LR, Martin F, Bailey RJ et al. A randomized, placebo-controlled, double-blind trial of mesalamine in the maintenance of remission of Crohn's disease. The Canadian Mesalamine for Remission of Crohn's disease Study group. *Gastroenterology* 1997; **112**: 1069–77.

419. Rutgeerts PJ, van Assche G, D'Haens G et al. Ornidazol for prophylaxis of post-operative Crohn's disease: final results of a placebo-controlled trial. *Gastroenterology* 2002; **122**: A135 (abstract).

420. Hellers G, Cortot A, Jewell D et al. Oral budesonide for prevention of postsurgical recurrence in Crohn's disease. The IOIBD Budesonide Study Group. *Gastroenterology* 1999; **116**: 294–300.

421. Kader HA, Raynor SC, Young R et al. Introduction of 6-mercaptopurine in Crohn's disease patients during the perioperative period: a preliminary evaluation of recurrence of disease. *J Paediatr Gastroenterol Nutr* 1997; **25**: 93–7.

422. Prantera C, Scribano ML, Falasco G et al. Ineffectiveness of probiotics in preventing recurrence after curative resection for Crohn's disease: a randomised controlled trial with *Lactobacillus GG*. *Gut* 2002; **51**: 405–9.

423. Rutgeerts PJ. Crohn's disease recurrence can be prevented after ileal resection. *Gut* 2002; **51**: 152–3.

424. Burnham WR, Lennard-Jones JC, Brooke B. Sexual problems among married ileostomists. *Gut* 1977; **18**: 673–7.

425. Wikland M, Jansson I, Asztely M et al. Gynaecological problems related to anatomical changes after conventional proctocolectomy and ileostomy. *Int J Colorect Dis* 1990; **5**: 49–52.

426. Moody G, Probert C, Srivastava E et al. Sexual dysfunction in women with Crohn's disease: a hidden problem. *Digestion* 1993; **52**: 179–83.

427. Lee ECG, Dowling BL. Perimuscular excision of the rectum for Crohn's disease and ulcerative colitis. *Br J Surg* 1972; **59**: 29–32.

428. Alstead EM. The pill: safe sex and Crohn's disease? *Gut* 1999; **45**: 165–6.

429. Rhodes JM, Cockel R, Allan RN et al. Colonic Crohn's disease and the use of oral contraception. *Br Med J* 1984; **288**: 595–6.
430. Bennett RA, Rubin PH, Present DH. Frequency of inflammatory bowel disease in offspring of couples both presenting with inflammatory bowel disease. *Gastroenterology* 1991; **100**: 1638–43.
431. Hudson M, Flett G, Sinclair TS et al. Fertility and pregnancy in inflammatory bowel disease. *Int J Gynaecol Obstetr* 1997; **58**: 229–37.
432. Alstead EM. How do fertility, pregnancy and lactation interact with inflammatory bowel disease? In: Rampton DS, ed. *Inflammatory Bowel Disease, Clinical Diagnosis and Management*. London: Martin Dunitz Ltd, 2000: 309–15.
433. Baird DD, Narendranathan M, Sandler RS. Increased risk of pre-term birth for women with inflammatory bowel disease. *Gastroenterology* 1990; **99**: 987–94.
434. Moody GA, Probert C, Jayanthi V et al. The effects of chronic ill health and treatment with sulphasalazine on fertility amongst men and women with inflammatory bowel disease in Leicestershire. *Int J Colorectal Dis* 1997; **12**: 220–4.
435. Farthing MJG, Dawson AM. Impaired semen quality in Crohn's disease – drugs, ill health or undernutrition? *Scand J Gastroenterol* 1983; **18**: 57–60.
436. Narendranathan M, Sandler RS, Suchindran M et al. Male infertility in inflammatory bowel disease. *J Clin Gastroenterol* 1989; **11**: 403–6.
437. Castiglione F, Pignata S, Morace F et al. Effect of pregnancy on the clinical course of a cohort of women with inflammatory bowel disease. *Ital J Gastroenterol* 1996; **28**: 199–204.
438. Moser MA, Okun NB, Mayes DC et al. Crohn's disease, pregnancy, and birth weight. *Am J Gastroenterol* 2000; **95**: 1021–6.
439. Miller JP. Inflammatory bowel disease in pregnancy: a review. *J R Soc Med* 1986; **79**: 221–9.
440. Morales M, Berney T, Jenny A et al. Crohn's disease as a risk factor for the outcome of pregnancy. *Hepatogastroenterology* 2000; **47**: 1595–8.
441. Fonager K, Sorensen HT, Olsen J et al. Pregnancy outcome for women with Crohn's disease: a follow-up study based on linkage between national registries. *Am J Gastroenterol* 1998; **93**: 2426–30.
442. Subhani JM, Hamilton MI. Review article. The management of inflammatory bowel disease during pregnancy. *Aliment Pharmacol Ther* 1998; **12**: 1039–53.
443. Cappell MS, Colonn VJ, Sidhom OA. A study of 10 medical centres of the safety and efficacy of 48 flexible sigmoidoscopies and 8 colonoscopies, during pregnancy with follow-up of fetal outcome and with comparison to control groups. *Dig Dis Sci* 1996; **41**: 2353–61.
444. Habal FM, Hui G, Greenberg GR. Oral 5-aminosalicylic acid for inflammatory bowel disease in pregnancy: safety and clinical course. *Gastroenterology* 1993; **105**: 1057–60.
445. Diav-Citrin O, Park YH, Veersuntharam G et al. The safety of mesalamine in human pregnancy: a prospective controlled cohort study. *Gastroenterology* 1998; **114**: 23–8.
446. Mogadem M, Dobbins WO, Korelitz BI et al. Pregnancy and inflammatory bowel disease: effect of sulphasalazine and corticosteroids on fetal outcome. *Gastroenterology* 1981; **80**: 72–6.
447. Piper JM, Mitchell EF, Ray WA. Prenatal use of metronidazole and birth defects: no association. *Obstet Gynecol* 1993; **82**: 348–52.
448. Connell W, Miller A. Treating inflammatory bowel disease during pregnancy: risks and safety of drug therapy. *Drug Safety* 1999; **21**: 311–23.
449. Loebstein R, Addis A, Ho E et al. Pregnancy outcome following gestational exposure to fluoroquinolones: a multicenter prospective controlled study. *Antimicrob Agents Chemother* 1998; **42**: 1336–9.

450. Srinivasan, R. Infliximab treatment and pregnancy outcome in active Crohn's disease. *Am J Gastroenterol* 2001; **96**: 2274–5.

451. Hill J, Clark A, Scott NA. Surgical treatment of acute manifestations of Crohn's disease during pregnancy. *J R Soc Med* 1997; **90**: 64–6.

452. Ilnyckyji A, Blanchard JF, Rawsthorne P et al. Perianal Crohn's disease and pregnancy: role of the mode of delivery. *Am J Gastroenterol* 1999; **94**: 3274–8.

453. Rogers RG, Katz VL. Course of Crohn's disease during pregnancy and its effect on pregnancy outcome: a retrospective review. *Am J Perinatol* 1995; **12**: 262–4.

454. Brandt LJ, Estabrook SG, Reinus JF. Results of a survey to evaluate whether vaginal delivery and episiotomy lead to perineal involvement in women with Crohn's disease. *Am J Gastroenterol* 1995; **90**: 1918–22.

455. Jarnerot G, Andersen S, Esbjorner E et al. Albumin reserve for binding in maternal and cord serum under treatment with sulphasalazine. *Scand J Gastroenterol* 1981; **16**: 1049–55.

456. Esbjorner E, Jarnerot G, Wranne L. Sulphasalazine and sulphapyridine levels in children to mothers treated with sulphasalazine during pregnancy and lactation. *Acta Paediatr Scand* 1987; **76**: 137–42.

457. Burakoff R, Opper F. Pregnancy and nursing. *Gastroenterol Clin North Am* 1995; **24**: 689–98.

458. Rayburn WF. Connective tissue disorders and pregnancy. Recommendations for prescribing. *J Reprod Med* 1998; **43**: 341–9.

459. Nwokolo CU, Tan WC, Andrews HA et al. Surgical resections in parous patients with distal ileal and colonic Crohn's disease. *Gut* 1994; **35**: 220–3.

460. Sawczenko A, Sandhu BK, Logan RF et al. Prospective survey of childhood inflammatory bowel disease in the British Isles. *Lancet* 2001; **357**: 1093–4.

461. Barton JR, Ferguson A. Clinical features, morbidity and mortality of Scottish children with inflammatory bowel disease. *Q J Med* 1990; **75**: 423–39.

462. Ballinger AB, Camacho-Hubner C, Croft NM. Growth failure and intestinal inflammation. *Q J Med* 2001; **94**: 121–5.

463. Bannerjee K, Croft NM, Babinska K et al. The influence of enteral feeding on growth factors, inflammation and nutrition in children with Crohn's disease. *Gastroenterology* 2000; **118**: A64 (abstract).

464. Tobin JM, Sinha B, Ramani P et al. Upper gastrointestinal mucosal disease in pediatric Crohn's disease and ulcerative colitis: a blinded, controlled study. *J Pediatr Gastroenterol Nutr* 2001; **32**: 443–8.

465. Davison SM, Chapman S, Murphy MS. 99mTc-HMPAO leucocyte scintigraphy fails to detect Crohn's disease in the proximal gastrointestinal tract. *Arch Dis Child* 2001; **85**: 43–6.

466. Tanner JM. *Growth at adolescence*, 2nd edition, Oxford, UK: Blackwell Scientific Publications, 1962.

467. Ghosh S, Drummond HE, Ferguson A. Neglect of growth and development in the clinical monitoring of children and teenagers with inflammatory bowel disease: review of case records. *Br Med J* 1998; **317**: 120–1.

468. Hildebrand H, Aronson S, Selvik G. Growth as a parameter of inflammation in Crohn's disease, using roentgen stereophotogrammetric analysis. *Acta Paediatr* 1994; **83**: 1070–5.

469. Hildebrand H, Karlberg J, Kristiansson B. Longitudinal growth in children and adolescents with inflammatory bowel disease. *J Pediatr Gastroenterol Nutr* 1994; **18**: 165–73.

470. Hyams JS, Ferry GD, Mandel FS et al. Development and validation of a pediatric Crohn's disease activity index. *J Pediatr Gastroenterol Nutr* 1991; **12**: 439–47.

471. Otley A, Loonen H, Parekh N et al. Assessing activity of pediatric Crohn's disease: which index to use? *Gastroenterology* 1999; **116**: 527–31.

472. Griffiths AM, Nicholas D, Smith C et al. Development of a quality-of-life index for pediatric inflammatory bowel disease: dealing with differences related to age and IBD type. *J Pediatr Gastroenterol Nutr* 1999; **28**: S46–52.

473. Richardson G, Griffiths AM, Miller V et al. Quality of life in inflammatory bowel disease: a cross-cultural comparison of English and Canadian children. *J Pediatr Gastroenterol Nutr* 2001; **32**: 573–8.

474. Axelsson C, Jarnum S. Assessment of the therapeutic value of an elemental diet in chronic inflammatory bowel disease. *Scand J Gastroenterol* 1977; **12**: 89–95.

475. Kirschner BS, Klich JR, Kalman SS et al. Reversal of growth retardation in Crohn's disease with therapy emphasising oral nutrition restitution. *Gastroenterology* 1981; **80**: 10–15.

476. O'Morain C, Segal AM, Levi AJ et al. Elemental diet in acute Crohn's disease. *Arch Dis Child* 1983; **58**: 44–7.

477. Sanderson IR, Udeen S, Davies PSW et al. Remission induced by an elemental diet in small bowel Crohn's disease. *Arch Dis Child* 1987; **61**: 123–7.

478. Thomas AG, Taylor F, Miller V. Dietary intake and nutritional treatment in childhood Crohn's disease. *J Pediatr Gastroenterol Nutr* 1993; **17**: 75–81.

479. Papadopoulou A, Rawashdeh MO, Brown GA et al. Remission following an elemental diet or prednisolone in Crohn's disease. *Acta Paediatr* 1995; **84**: 79–83.

480. Ruuska T, Savilahti E, Maki M et al. Exclusive whole protein enteral diet versus prednisolone in the treatment of acute Crohn's disease in children. *J Pediatr Gastroenterol Nutr* 1994; **19**: 175–80.

481. Bannerjee K, Croft NM, Camacho-Hubner C et al. Anti-inflammatory and pro-growth effects precede nutritional changes during enteral feeding in active Crohn's disease. *J Pediatr Gastroenterol Nutr* 2000; **31**: S274 (abstract).

482. Heuschkel RB, Walker-Smith JA. Enteral nutrition in inflammatory bowel disease of childhood. *J Parenter Enteral Nutr* 1999; **23**: S29–32.

483. Beattie RM, Bentsen BS, MacDonald TT. Childhood Crohn's disease and the efficacy of enteral diets. *Nutrition* 1998; **14**: 345–50.

484. Randell T, Murphy MS. Evaluation of elemental therapy as a long term strategy for managing Crohn's disease in childhood. *Arch Dis Child* 2002; **84**: A4 (abstract).

485. Ali E, Crouchman P, Meadows N et al. Outcome of enteral feeding for newly diagnosed Crohn's disease. *Gut* 2002; **50**: A71–72 (abstract).

486. Sandhu BK, Knight C, Matary W. Long-term outcome of elemental diet as primary therapy for pediatric Crohn's disease. *Gastroenterology* 2002; **122**: A12 (abstract).

487. Belli DC, Seidman E, Bouthillier L et al. Chronic intermittent elemental diet improves growth failure in children with Crohn's disease. *Gastroenterology* 1988; **94**: 603–10.

488. Polk DB, Hattner JA, Kerner JA Jr. Improved growth and disease activity after intermittent administration of a defined formula diet in children with Crohn's disease. *J Parenter Enteral Nutr* 1992; **16**: 499–504.

489. Wilschanski M, Sherman P, Pencharz P et al. Supplementary enteral nutrition maintains remission in paediatric Crohn's disease. *Gut* 1996; **38**: 543–48.

490. Cosgrove M, Jenkins HR. Experience of percutaneous endoscopic gastrostomy in children with Crohn's disease. *Arch Dis Child* 1997; **76**: 141–3.

491. Soyka LF. Alternate-day corticosteroid therapy. *Adv Pediatr* 1972; **19**: 47–70.

492. Zachos M, Tondeur M, Griffiths AM. Enteral nutritional therapy for inducing remission of Crohn's disease. Oxford: *The Cochrane Library*, The Cochrane Collaborations; Update Software, 2002.

493. Kundhal P, Zachos M, Holmes JL et al. Controlled ileal release budesonide in pediatric Crohn disease: efficacy and effect on growth. *J Pediatr Gastroenterol Nutr* 2001; **33**: 75–80.

494. Levine A, Broide E, Stein M et al. Evaluation of oral budesonide for treatment of mild and moderate exacerbations of Crohn's disease in children. *J Pediatr* 2002; **140**: 75–80.

495. Escher JC, Lindquist B, Hildebrand H et al. Budesonide capsules versus prednisolone in children with active Crohn's disease: results of a European multicentre study. *Gastroenterology* 2002; **122**: A12 (abstract).

496. Cowan FJ, Warner JT, Dunstan FD et al. Inflammatory bowel disease and predisposition to osteopenia. *Arch Dis Child* 1997; **76**: 325–9.

497. Boot AM, Krenning P, de Muinck Keizer-Schrama SMPF. Bone mineral density and nutritional status in children with chronic inflammatory bowel disease. *Gut* 1998; **42**: 188–94.

498. Ho J, Akanle OA, Savage MO et al. Bone mineral density at diagnosis in paediatric inflammatory bowel disease. *J Pediatr Gastroenterol Nutr* 2002; **34**: 451.

499. Griffiths A, Koletzko S, Sylvester F et al. Slow-release 5-aminosalicylic acid therapy in children with small intestinal Crohn's disease. *J Pediatr Gastroenterol Nutr* 1993; **17**: 186–92.

500. Ferry GD, Kirschner BS, Grand RJ et al. Olsalazine versus sulfasalazine in mild to moderate childhood ulcerative colitis: results of the Pediatric Gastroenterology Collaborative Research Group Clinical Trial. *J Pediatr Gastroenterol Nutr* 1993; **17**: 32–8.

501. Markowitz J, Grancher K, Kohn N et al. A multicenter trial of 6-mercaptopurine and prednisone in children with newly diagnosed Crohn's disease. *Gastroenterology* 2000; **119**: 895–902.

502. Casson DH, Davies SE, Thomson MA et al. Low-dose intravenous azathioprine may be effective in the management of acute fulminant colitis complicating inflammatory bowel disease. *Aliment Pharmacol Ther* 1999; **13**: 891–5.

503. Mack DR, Young R, Kaufman SS et al. Methotrexate in patients with Crohn's disease after 6-mercaptopurine. *J Pediatr* 1998; **132**: 830–5.

504. Mahdi G, Israel DM, Hassall E. Cyclosporine and 6-mercaptopurine for active, refractory Crohn's colitis in children. *Am J Gastroenterol* 1996; **91**: 1355–9.

505. Ramakrishna J, Langhans N, Calenda K et al. Combined use of cyclosporine and azathioprine or 6-mercaptopurine in pediatric inflammatory bowel disease. *J Pediatr Gastroenterol Nutr* 1996; **22**: 296–302.

506. Nicholls S, Domizio P, Williams CB et al. Cyclosporin as initial treatment for Crohn's disease. *Arch Dis Child* 1994; **71**: 243–7.

507. Bousvaros A, Kirschner BS, Werlin SL et al. Oral tacrolimus treatment of severe colitis in children. *J Pediatr* 2000; **137**: 794–9.

508. Breese EJ, Michie CA, Nicholls SW et al. Tumor necrosis factor alpha-producing cells in the intestinal mucosa of children with inflammatory bowel disease. *Gastroenterology* 1994; **106**: 1455–66.

509. Hyams JS, Markowitz J, Wyllie R. Use of infliximab in the treatment of Crohn's disease in children and adolescents. *J Pediatr* 2000; **137**: 192–6.

510. Facchini S, Candusso M, Martelossi S et al. Efficacy of long-term treatment with thalidomide in children and young adults with Crohn's disease: preliminary results. *J Pediatr Gastroenterol Nutr* 2001; **32**: 178–81.

511. Russell RK, Richardson N, Wilson DC. Systemic absorption with complications during topical tacrolimus treatment for orofacial Crohn disease. *J Pediatr Gastroenterol Nutr* 2001; **32**: 207–8.

512. Gupta P, Andrew H, Kirschner BS et al. Is lactobacillus GG helpful in children with Crohn's disease? Results of a preliminary, open-label study. *J Pediatr Gastroenterol Nutr* 2000; **31**: 453–7.

513. Farmer RG, Michener WM. Prognosis of Crohn's disease with onset in childhood or adolescence. *Dig Dis Sci* 1979; **24**: 752–7.

514. Davies G, Evans CM, Shand WS et al. Surgery for Crohn's disease in childhood: influence of site of disease and operative procedure on outcome. *Br J Surg* 1990; **77**: 891–4.

515. Besnard M, Jaby O, Mougenot JF et al. Postoperative outcome of Crohn's disease in 30 children. *Gut* 1998; **43**: 634–8.

516. Hyams JS, Moore RE, Leichtner AM et al. Longitudinal assessment of type I procollagen in children with inflammatory bowel disease subjected to surgery. *J Pediatr Gastroenterol Nutr* 1989; **8**: 68–74.

517. McLain BI, Davidson PM, Stokes KB et al. Growth after gut resection for Crohn's disease. *Arch Dis Child* 1990; **65**: 760–2.

518. Lim S, Dohil R, Meadows N et al. Treatment of orofacial and ileo-colonic Crohn's disease with total enteral nutrition. *J R Soc Med* 1998; **91**: 489–90.

519. Kleist P. Pediatric drug development. *App Clin Trials* 2002; **xx**: 40–8.

520. Han PD, Burke A, Baldassano RN et al. Nutrition and inflammatory bowel disease. *Gastroenterol Clin North Am* 1999; **28**: 423–43.

521. Durnin JV, Womersley J. Body fat assessed from total body density and its estimation from skinfold thickness: measurements on 481 men and women aged from 16 to 72 years. *Br J Nutr* 1974; **32**: 77–97.

522. Martin S, Neale G, Elia M. Factors affecting maximum momentary grip strength. *Hum Nutr Clin Nutr* 1985; **39**: 137–47.

523. Harris JA, Benedict FG. A biometric study of basal metabolism in man. Carnegie Institute Publication No. 279. Washington: Carnegie Institute, 1919.

524. Elia M. Artificial nutritional support. *Med Int* 1990; **82**: 3392–6.

525. Anstee QM, Forbes A. The safe use of percutaneous gastrostomy for enteral nutrition in patients with Crohn's disease. *Eur J Gastroenterol Hepatol* 2000; **12**: 1089–93.

526. Matsui T, Ueki M, Yamada M et al. Indications and options of nutritional treatment for Crohn's disease. A comparison of elemental and polymeric diets. *J Gastroenterol* 1995; **30** (Suppl 8): 95–7.

527. Jeppesen PB, Langholz E. Mortensen PB. Quality of life in patients receiving home parenteral nutrition. *Gut* 1999; **44**: 844–52.

528. Solomon SM, Kirby DF. The refeeding syndrome: a review. *J Parenter Enteral Nutr* 1990; **14**: 90–7.

529. Crook MA, Hally V, Panteli JV. The importance of the refeeding syndrome. *Nutrition* 2001; **17**: 632–7.

530. Nightingale JMD. Management of patients with a short bowel. *World J Gastroenterol* 2001; **7**: 741–51.

531. Anonymous. AGA technical review on short bowel syndrome and intestinal transplantation. *Gastroenterology* 2003; **124**. 1111–34.

532. McNeil NI. The contribution of the large intestine to energy supplies in man. *Am J Clin Nutr* 1984; **39**: 338–42.

533. Nightingale JM, Lennard-Jones JE, Walker ER et al. Jejunal efflux in short bowel syndrome. *Lancet* 1990; **336**: 765–8.

534. Temperley JM, Stagg BH, Wyllie JH. Disappearance of gastrin and pentagastrin in the portal circulation. *Gut* 1971; **12**: 372–6.

535. Fielding JF, Cooke WT, Williams JA. Gastric acid secretion in Crohn's disease in relation to disease activity and bowel resection. *Lancet* 1971; **i**: 1106–7.

536. Nightingale JMD, Kamm MA, van der Sijp JRB et al. Gastrointestinal hormones in the short bowel syndrome. PYY may be the 'colonic brake' to gastric emptying. *Gut* 1996; **39**: 267–72.

537. Booth CC, Mollin DL. The site of absorption of vitamin B_{12} in man. *Lancet* 1959; **i**: 18–21.

538. Pironi L, Pagnelli GM, Miglioli M et al. Morphologic and cytoproliferative patterns of duodenal mucosa in two patients after long-term total parenteral

nutrition: changes with oral refeeding and relation to intestinal resection. *J Parenter Enteral Nutr* 1994; **18**: 351–4.

539. Carbonnel F, Cosnes J, Chevret S et al. The role of anatomic factors in nutritional autonomy after extensive small bowel resection. *J Parenter Enteral Nutr* 1996; **20**: 275–80.

540. Nightingale JMD, Walsh N, Bullock ME et al. Comparison of three simple methods for the detection of malnutrition. *J R Soc Med* 1996; **89**: 144–8.

541. King RFGJ, Norton T, Hill GL. A double-blind crossover study of the effect of loperamide hydrochloride and codeine phosphate on ileostomy output. *Aust NZ J Surg* 1982; **52**: 121–4.

542. Nightingale JMD, Walker ER, Farthing MJG et al. Effect of omeprazole on intestinal output in the short bowel syndrome. *Aliment Pharmacol Ther* 1991; **5**: 405–12.

543. Dharmsathaphorn K, Gorelick FS, Sherwin RS et al. Somatostatin decreases diarrhoea in patients with the short bowel syndrome. *J Clin Gastroenterol* 1982; **4**: 521–4.

544. Cooper JC, Williams NS, King RFGJ et al. Effects of a long acting somatostatin analogue in patients with severe ileostomy diarrhoea. *Br J Surg* 1986; **73**: 128–31.

545. Kayne LH, Lee DB. Intestinal magnesium absorption. *Miner Electrolyte Metab* 1993; **19**: 210–17.

546. Hanna S, McIntyre I. The influence of aldosterone on magnesium metabolism. *Lancet* 1960; **ii**: 348–50.

547. Zofkova I, Kancheva RL. The relationship between magnesium and calciotropic hormones. *Magnes Res* 1995; **8**: 77–84.

548. Fukumoto S, Matsumoto T, Tanaka Y et al. Renal magnesium wasting in a patient with short bowel syndrome with magnesium deficiency: effect of 1 alpha-hydroxyvitamin D3 treatment. *J Clin Endocrinol Metab* 1987; **65**: 1301–4.

549. Press M, Hartop PJ, Prottey C. Correction of essential fatty-acid deficiency in man by the cutaneous application of sunflower-seed oil. *Lancet* 1974; **i**: 598–9.

550. Rannem T, Ladefoged K, Hylander E et al. Selenium depletion in patients on home parenteral nutrition. The effect of selenium supplementation. *Biol Trace Elem Res* 1993; **39**: 81–90.

551. Wolman SL, Anderson GH, Marliss EB et al. Zinc in total parenteral nutrition: requirements and metabolic effects. *Gastroenterology* 1979; **76**: 458–67.

552. Howard L, Ament M, Fleming CR et al. Current use and clinical outcome of home parenteral and enteral nutrition therapies in the United States. *Gastroenterology* 1995; **109**: 355–65.

553. Spiller RC, Brown ML, Phillips SF. Decreased fluid tolerance, accelerated transit, and abnormal motility of the human colon induced by oleic acid. *Gastroenterology* 1986; **91**: 100–7.

554. Jeppesen PB, Mortensen PB. Colonic digestion and absorption of energy from carbohydrates and medium-chain fat in small bowel failure. *J Parenter Enteral Nutr* 1999; **23**(Suppl 5): S101–5.

555. Nordgaard I, Hansen BS, Mortensen PB. Importance of colonic support for energy absorption as small-bowel failure proceeds. *Am J Clin Nutr* 1996; **64**: 222–31.

556. Ovesen L, Chu R, Howard L. The influence of dietary fat on jejunostomy output in patients with severe short bowel syndrome. *Am J Clin Nutr* 1983; **38**: 270–7.

557. Brophy DF, Ford SL, Crouch MA. Warfarin resistance in a patient with short bowel syndrome. *Pharmacotherapy* 1998; **18**: 646–9.

558. Ehrenpreis ED, Guerriero S, Nogueras JJ et al. Malabsorption of digoxin tablets, gel caps, and elixir in a patient with an end jejunostomy. *Ann Pharmacother* 1994; **28**: 1239–40.

559. Sustento-Reodica N, Ruiz P, Rogers A et al. Recurrent Crohn's disease in transplanted bowel. *Lancet* 1997; **349**: 688–91.

560. Binder V. Cancer in inflammatory bowel disease: how common is it and how can it be prevented? In: Rampton DS, ed. *Inflammatory Bowel Disease, Clinical Diagnosis and Management*. London: Martin Dunitz Ltd, 2000, 265–76.

561. Gillen CD, Walmsley RS, Prior P et al. Ulcerative colitis and Crohn's disease: a comparison of the colorectal cancer risk in extensive colitis. *Gut* 1994; **35**: 1590–2.

562. Bernstein CN, Blanchard JF, Kliewer E et al. Cancer risk in patients with inflammatory bowel disease: a population-based study. *Cancer* 2001; **91**: 854–62.

563. Greenstein AJ. Cancer in inflammatory bowel disease. *Mt Sinai J Med* 2000; **67**: 227–40.

564. Pohl C, Hombach A, Kruis W. Chronic inflammatory bowel disease and cancer. *Hepatogastroenterology* 2000; **47**: 57–70.

565. Askling J, Dickman PW, Karlen P et al. Family history as a risk factor for colorectal cancer in inflammatory bowel disease. *Gastroenterology* 2001; **120**: 1356–62.

566. Sigel JE, Petras RE, Lashner BA et al. Intestinal adenocarcinoma in Crohn's disease: a report of 30 cases with a focus on coexisting dysplasia. *Am J Surg Pathol* 1999; **23**: 651–5.

567. Lashner BA, Heidenreich PA, Su GL et al. Effect of folate supplementation on the incidence of dysplasia and cancer in chronic ulcerative colitis. *Gastroenterology* 1989; **97**: 255–9.

568. Moody GA, Jayanthi V, Probert CSJ et al. Long-term therapy with sulphasalazine protects against colorectal cancer in ulcerative colitis: a retrospective study of colorectal cancer risk and compliance with treatment in Leicestershire. *Eur J Gastroenterol* 1996; **8**: 1179–83.

569. Greenstein AJ, Sachar DB, Smith H et al. Patterns of neoplasia in Crohn's disease and ulcerative colitis. *Cancer* 1980; **46**: 403–7.

570. Hawker PC, Gyde SN, Thompson H et al. Adenocarcinoma of the small intestine complicating Crohn's disease. *Gut* 1982; **23**: 188–93.

571. Ribeiro MB, Greenstein AJ, Heimann TM et al. Adenocarcinoma of the small intestine in Crohn's disease. *Surg Gynecol Obstet* 1991; **173**: 343–9.

572. Jaskowiak NT, Michelassi F. Adenocarcinoma at a strictureplasty site in Crohn's disease: report of a case. *Dis Colon Rectum* 2001; **44**: 284–7.

573. Yamamoto T, Allan RN, Keighley MR. Long-term outcome of surgical management for diffuse jejunoileal Crohn's disease. *Surgery* 2001; **129**: 96–102.

574. Frisch M, Johansen C. Anal carcinoma in inflammatory bowel disease. *Br J Cancer* 2000; **83**: 89–90.

575. Buchman AL, Ament ME, Doty J. Development of squamous cell carcinoma in chronic perineal sinus and wounds in Crohn's disease. *Am J Gastroenterol* 1991; **86**: 1829–32.

576. Veloso FT, Carvalho J, Magro F. Immune-related systemic manifestations of inflammatory bowel disease. A prospective study of 792 patients. *J Clin Gastroenterol* 1996; **23**: 29–34.

577. Lamers CBHW. Extraintestinal manifestations and complications of inflammatory bowel disease. In: Rampton DS, ed. *Inflammatory Bowel Disease, Clinical Diagnosis and Management*. London: Martin Dunitz Ltd, 2000, 295–307.

578. Bernstein CN, Blanchard JF, Rawsthorne P et al. The prevalence of extraintestinal diseases in inflammatory bowel disease: a population-based study. *Am J Gastroenterol* 2001; **96**: 1116–22.

579. Orchard TR, Wordsworth BP, Jewell DP. Peripheral arthropathies in inflammatory bowel disease: their articular distribution and natural history. *Gut* 1998; **42**: 387–91.

580. Orchard TR, Thiyagaraja S, Welsh KI et al. Clinical phenotype is related to HLA genotype in the peripheral arthropathies of inflammatory bowel disease. *Gastroenterology* 2000; **118**: 274–8.

581. Mahadevan U, Loftus EV, Tremaine WJ et al. Safety of selective COX-2 inhibitors in inflammatory bowel disease. *Am J Gastroenterol* 2002; **97**: 910–14.

582. Mielants H, Veys EM. HLA-B27 related arthritis and bowel inflammation. Part 1. Sulphasalazine (salazopyrin) in HLA-B27 related reactive arthritis. *J Rheumatol* 1985; **12**: 287–93.

583. Orchard TR, Jewell DP. The importance of ileocaecal integrity in the arthritic complications of Crohn's disease. *Inflamm Bowel Dis* 1999; **5**: 92–7.

584. Hasko G, Sazbo C, Nemeth ZH et al. Sulphasalazine inhibits macrophage activation: inhibitory effects on inducible nitric oxide synthase expression, interleukin-12 production and major histocompatibility complex II expression. *Immunology* 2001; **103**: 473–8.

585. Kitis G, Thompson H, Allan RN. Finger clubbing in inflammatory bowel disease: its prevalence and pathogenesis. *Br Med J* 1979; **ii**: 825–8.

586. Soukiasian S, Foster CS, Raizman MB. Treatment strategies for scleritis and uveitis associated with inflammatory bowel disease. *Am J Ophthalmol* 1994; **118**: 601–11.

587. Salmon JF, Wright JP, Murray AD. Ocular inflammation in Crohn's disease. *Ophthalmology* 1991; **98**: 480–4.

588. Orchard TR, Chua CN, Ahmad T et al. Uveitis and erythema nodosum in inflammatory bowel disease: clinical features and the role of HLA genes. *Gastroenterology* 2002; **123**: 714–18.

589. Verbraak FD, Schreinemachers MC, Tiller A et al. Prevalence of subclinical anterior uveitis in a patients with inflammatory bowel disease. *Br J Ophthalmol* 2001; **85**: 219–21.

590. Levitt MD, Ritchie JK, Lennard-Jones JE et al. Pyoderma gangrenosum in inflammatory bowel disease. *Br J Surg* 1991; **78**: 676–8.

591. Carp JM, Onuma E, Das K et al. Intravenous cyclosporin therapy in the treatment of pyoderma gangrenosum secondary to inflammatory bowel disease. *Cutis* 1997; **60**: 135–8.

592. Dwarakanath AD, Yu LG, Brookes C et al. 'Sticky' neutrophils, pathergic arthritis, and response to heparin in pyoderma gangrenosum complicating ulcerative colitis. *Gut* 1995; **37**: 585–8.

593. Tan MH, Gordon M, Lebwohl O et al. Improvement of pyoderma gangrenosum and psoriasis associated with Crohn's disease with anti-tumor necrosis factor alpha monoclonal antibody. *Arch Dermatol* 2001; **137**: 930–3.

594. Rasmussen HH, Fallingborg JF, Mortensen PB et al. Hepatobiliary dysfunction and primary sclerosing cholangitis in patients with Crohn's disease. *Scand J Gastroenterol* 1997; **32**: 604–10.

595. Chapman RW. Hepatobiliary disorders. In: Rampton DS, ed. *Inflammatory Bowel Disease, Clinical Diagnosis and Management*. London, UK: Martin Dunitz Ltd, 2000, 277–95.

596. Chapman RW, Arborgh BA, Rhodes JM et al. Primary sclerosing cholangitis – a review of its clinical features, cholangiography and hepatic histology. *Gut* 1980; **21**: 870–7.

597. Seibold F, Weber P, Schoning A et al. Neutrophil antibodies (pANCA) in chronic liver disease and inflammatory bowel disease: do they react with different antigens? *Eur J Gastroenterol Hepatol* 1996; **8**: 1095–100.

598. Ferrara C, Valeri G, Salvolini L et al. Magnetic resonance cholangiopancreatography in primary sclerosing cholangitis in children. *Pediatr Radiol* 2002; **32**: 413–17.

599. Lindor KD. Ursodiol for primary sclerosing cholangitis. Mayo Primary Sclerosing Cholangitis–Ursodeoxycholic Acid Study Group. *N Engl J Med* 1997; **336**: 691–5.
600. Mitchell SA, Bansi DS, Hunt N et al. A preliminary trial of high-dose ursodeoxycholic acid in primary sclerosing cholangitis. *Gastroenterology* 2001; **121**: 900–7.
601. Befeler AS, Lissoos TW, Schiano TD et al. Clinical course and management of inflammatory bowel disease after liver transplantation. *Transplantation* 1998; **65**: 393–6.
602. Tung BY, Emond MJ, Haggitt RC et al. Ursodiol use is associated with lower prevalence of colonic neoplasia in patients with ulcerative colitis and primary sclerosing cholangitis. *Ann Intern Med* 2001; **134**: 89–95.
603. Berman MD, Falchuk KR, Trey C. Carcinoma of the biliary tree complicating Crohn's disease. *Dig Dis Sci* 1980; **25**: 795–7.
604. Choi PM, Nugent FW, Zelig MP et al. Cholangiocarcinoma and Crohn's disease. *Dig Dis Sci* 1994; **39**: 667–70.
605. Ponsioen CY, Vtouenraets SM, van Milligen de Wit AW et al. Value of brush cytology for dominant strictures in primary sclerosing cholangitis. *Endoscopy* 1999; **31**: 305–9.
606. Broome U, Olsson R, Loof L et al. Natural history and prognostic factors in 305 Swedish patients with primary sclerosing cholangitis. *Gut* 1996; **38**: 610–15.
607. Steiber AL, Marino IR, Iwatsuki S et al. Cholangiocarcinoma in sclerosing cholangitis: the role of liver transplantation. *Int J Surg* 1989; **74**: 1–3.
608. van Leeuwen DJ, Reeders JW. Primary sclerosing cholangitis and cholangiocarcinoma as a diagnostic and therapeutic dilemma. *Ann Oncol* 1999; **10**(Suppl 4): 89–93.
609. Olsson R, Hulten L. Concurrence of ulcerative colitis and chronic active hepatitis. Clinical courses and results of colectomy. *Scand J Gastroenterol* 1975; **10**: 331–5.
610. Kangas E, Lehmusto P, Matikainen M. Gallstones in Crohn's disease. *Hepatogastroenterology* 1990; **37**: 83–7.
611. Murray FE, McNicholas M, Stack W et al. Impaired fatty meal stimulated gall bladder contractivity in patients with Crohn's disease. *Clin Sci* 1993; **83**: 689–93.
612. Suhr O, Danielsson A, Nyhlin H et al. Bile acid malabsorption demonstrated by SeHCAT in chronic diarrhoea, with special reference to the impact of cholecystectomy. *Scand J Gastroenterol* 1988; **23**: 1187–94.
613. Perret AD, Higgins H, Johnston HH et al. The liver in Crohn's disease. *Q J Med* 1971; **40**: 187–209.
614. Greenstein AJ, Sachar DB, Panday AK et al. Amyloidosis and inflammatory bowel disease. A 50-year experience with 25 patients. *Medicine* 1992; **71**: 261–70.
615. Lovat LB, Madhoo S, Pepys MB et al. Long-term survival in systemic amyloid A amyloidosis complicating Crohn's disease. *Gastroenterology* 1997; **112**: 1362–5.
616. Rankin GB. Extraintestinal manifestations of inflammatory bowel disease. *Med Clin North Am* 1990; **74**: 39–50.
617. Earnest DL. Enteric hyperoxaluria. *Adv Intern Med* 1979; **24**: 407–27.
618. Rampton DS, Sarner M. Enteric and other secondary hyperoxalurias. In: Rose GA, ed. *Oxalate Metabolism in Relation to Urinary Stone*, London: Springer-Verlag, 1988, 103–20.
619. Caspary WF, Tonissen J, Lankisch PG. 'Enteral' hyperoxaluria. Effect of cholestyramine, calcium, neomycin, and bile acids on intestinal oxalate absorption in man. *Acta Hepatogastroenterol* 1977; **24**: 193–200.
620. Compston JE. Review article: osteoporosis, corticosteroids and inflammatory bowel disease. *Aliment Pharmacol Ther* 1995; **9**: 237–50.
621. Bernstein CN, Blanchard JF, Leslie W et al. The incidence of fracture among patients with inflammatory bowel disease. A population-based cohort study. *Ann Intern Med* 2000; **133**: 795–9.

622. Loftus EV Jr, Crowson CS, Sandborn WJ et al. Long term fracture risk in patients with Crohn's disease: a population-based study in Olmsted County, Minnesota. *Gastroenterology* 2002; **123**: 468–75.
623. Bjarnason I, Macpherson A, Mackintosh C et al. Reduced bone density in patients with inflammatory bowel disease. *Gut* 1997; **40**: 228–33.
624. Arden NK, Cooper C. Osteoporosis in patients with inflammatory bowel disease. *Gut* 2002; **50**: 9–10.
625. Lukert BP, Raisz LG. Glucocorticoid-induced osteoporosis: pathogenesis and management. *Ann Intern Med* 1990; **112**: 352–64.
626. Nemetz A, Tóth M, Garciá-González MA et al. Allelic variation of the interleukin 1β gene is associated with decreased bone mass in patients with inflammatory bowel disease. *Gut* 2001; **49**: 644–9.
627. Bousser MG, Canard J, Kittner S et al. Recommendations on the risk of ischaemic stroke associated with the use of combined oral contraceptives and hormone replacement therapy in women with migraine. The International Headache Society Task Force on combined oral contraceptives and hormone replacement therapy. *Cephalgia* 2000; **20**: 155–6.
628. Mannucci PM. Venous thromboembolism and hormone replacement therapy. *Eur J Intern Med* 2001; **12**: 478–83.
629. Psaty BM, Smith NL, Lemaitre RN et al. Hormone replacement therapy, pro-thrombotic mutations, and the risk of incident non-fatal myocardial infarction in postmenopausal women. *JAMA* 2001; **285**: 906–13.
630. Cauley JA, Seeley DG, Ensrud K et al. Estrogen replacement therapy and fractures in older women. *Ann Intern Med* 1995; **122**: 9–16.
631. Chen CL, Weiss NS, Newcomb P et al. Hormone replacement therapy in relation to breast cancer. *JAMA* 2002; **287**: 734–41.
632. Orwoll ES, Klein RF. Osteoporosis in men. *Endocr Rev* 1995; **16**: 87–116.
633. Younes H, Farhat G, Fuleihan Gel-H. Efficacy and tolerability of cyclical intravenous pamidronate in patients with low bone mass. *J Clin Densitom* 2002; **5**: 143–9.
634. Cremers S, Sparidans R, Den HJ et al. A pharmacokinetic and pharmacodynamic model for intravenous bisphosphonate (pamidronate) in osteoporosis. *Eur J Clin Pharmacol* 2002; **57**: 883–90.
635. Woo T, Adachi JD. Role of bisphosphonates and calcitonin in the prevention and treatment of osteoporosis. *Best Pract Res Clin Rheumatol* 2001; **15**: 469–81.
636. Haderslev KV, Tjellesen L, Sorensen HA et al. Alendronate increases lumbar spine bone mineral density in patients with Crohn's disease. *Gastroenterology* 2000; **119**: 639–46.
637. Eastell R. Management of glucocorticoid-induced osteoporosis. *J Intern Med* 1995; **237**: 439–47.
638. Gasche C. Anemia in IBD: the overlooked villain. *Inflamm Bowel Dis* 2000; **6**: 142–50.
639. Bartels U, Pedersen NS, Jarnum S. Iron absorption and serum ferritin in chronic inflammatory bowel disease. *Scand J Gastroenterol* 1978; **13**: 649–56.
640. Provan D. Mechanisms and management of iron deficiency anaemia. *Br J Haematol* 1999; **105**(Suppl 1): 19–26.
641. de Silva AD, Mylonaki M, Kampton D3. Oral iron therapy in inflammatory bowel disease: usage, tolerance and efficacy. *Inflamm Bowel Dis* 2003 (in press).
642. Gasche C, Dejaco C, Waldhoer T et al. Intravenous iron and erythropoietin for anemia associated with Crohn's disease. *Ann Int Med* 1997; **126**: 782–7.
643. Schreiber S, Howaldt S, Schnoor M et al. Recombinant erythropoietin for the treatment of anemia in inflammatory bowel disease. *N Engl J Med* 1996; **334**: 619–23.

644. Gasche C, Waldoer T, Feichtenschlager T et al. Prediction of response to iron sucrose in inflammatory bowel disease-associated anaemia. *Am J Gastroenterol* 2001; **96**: 2382–7.

645. Webberley MJ, Hart MT, Melikian V. Thromboembolism in inflammatory bowel disease: role of platelets. *Gut* 1993; **34**: 247–51.

646. Warren S, Sommers SC. Pathogenesis of ulcerative colitis. *Am J Pathol* 1949; **25**: 657–74.

647. Sloan WP, Bargen JA, Gage RP. Life histories of patients with chronic ulcerative colitis: a review of 2000 cases. *Gastroenterology* 1950; **16**: 25–38.

648. Harries AD, Fitzsimons E, Fifield R et al. Platelet count: a simple measure of activity in Crohn's disease. *Br Med J* 1983; **286**: 1476.

649. Collins CE, Cahill MR, Newland AC et al. Platelets circulate in an activated state in inflammatory bowel disease. *Gastroenterology* 1994; **106**: 840–5.

650. Liebman HA, Kashani N, Sutherland D et al. The factor V Leiden mutation increases the risk of venous thrombosis in patients with inflammatory bowel disease. *Gastroenterology* 1998; **115**: 830–4.

651. Jackson LM, O'Gorman PJ, O'Connell J et al. Thrombosis in inflammatory bowel disease: clinical setting, procoagulant profile and factor V Leiden. *Q J Med* 1997; **90**: 183–8.

652. Aadland E, Odegaard OR, Roseth A et al. Free protein S deficiency in patients with chronic inflammatory bowel disease. *Scand J Gastroenterol* 1992; **27**: 957–60.

653. Novacek G, Miehsler W, Kapiotis S et al. Thromboembolism and resistance to activated protein C in patients with inflammatory bowel disease. *Am J Gastroenterol* 1999; **94**: 685–90.

654. Wakefield AL, Sawyer AM, Hudson M et al. Smoking, the oral contraceptive pill, and Crohn's disease. *Dig Dis Sci* 1991; **36**: 1147–50.

655. Casati J, Toner BB, de Rooy EC et al. Concerns of patients with inflammatory bowel disease. A review of emerging issues. *Dig Dis Sci* 2000; **45**: 26–31.

656. de Rooy EC, Toner BB, Maunder RG et al. Concerns of patients with inflammatory bowel disease: results from a clinical population. *Am J Gastroenterol* 2001; **96**: 1816–21.

657. Engstrom I. Inflammatory bowel disease in children and adolescents: mental health and family functioning. *J Pediatr Gastroenterol Nutr* 1999; **28**: S28–33.

658. Rickards H, Prendergast M, Booth I. Psychiatric presentation of Crohn's disease. Diagnostic delay and increased morbidity. *Br J Psychiatry* 1994; **164**: 256–61.

659. Mansfield JC, Tanner AR, Bramble MG. Information for patients about inflammatory bowel disease. *J R Coll Physicians Lond* 1997; **31**: 184–7.

660. Maunder RG, de Rooy EC, Toner BB et al. Health-related concerns of people who receive psychological support for inflammatory bowel disease. *Can J Gastroenterol* 1997; **11**: 681–5.

661. Moser G, Tillinger W, Sachs G et al. Disease-related worries and concerns: a study on out-patients with inflammatory bowel disease. *Eur J Gastroenterol Hepatol* 1995; **7**: 853–8.

662. Verma S, Tsai HH, Giaffer MH. Does better disease-related education improve quality of life? A survey of IBD patients. *Dig Dis Sci* 2001; **46**: 865–9.

663. Brook A, Bingley J. The contribution of psychotherapy to patients with disorders of the gut. *Health Trends* 1991; **23**: 83–5.

664. de Boer AG, Sprangers MA, Bartelsman JF et al. Predictors of health care utilization in patients with inflammatory bowel disease: a longitudinal study. *Eur J Gastroenterol Hepatol* 1998; **10**: 783–9.

665. Rabbett H, Elbadri A, Thwaites R et al. Quality of life in children with Crohn's disease. *J Pediatr Gastroenterol Nutr* 1996; **23**: 528–33.

666. Mayberry JF. The patient in the community: psycho-social and practical issues. In: Rampton DS, ed. *Inflammatory Bowel Disease, Clinical Diagnosis and Management*. London: Martin Dunitz Ltd, 2000, 253–62.

667. Bernstein CN, Kraut A, Blanchard JF et al. The relationship between inflammatory bowel disease and socioeconomic variables. *Am J Gastroenterol* 2001; **96**: 2117–25.

668. Mayberry MK, Probert C, Srivastava E et al. Perceived discrimination in education and employment by people with Crohn's disease: a case-control study of educational achievement and employment. *Gut* 1992; **33**: 312–14.

669. Ferguson A, Sedgewick DM, Drummond J. Morbidity of juvenile onset inflammatory bowel disease: effects on education and employment in early adult life. *Gut* 1994; **35**: 665–8.

670. Probert CSJ, Mayberry M, Mayberry JF. Education and young people with inflammatory bowel disease. *J R Soc Health* 1992; **112**: 112–13.

671. Mayberry MK, Mayberry JF. An information booklet for schools to help teachers deal with students with inflammatory bowel disease. *J Clin Nursing* 1993; **2**: 19–22.

672. Moody GA, Probert CSJ, Jayanthi V et al. The attitude of employers to people with inflammatory bowel disease. *Soc Sci Med* 1992; **34**: 459–60.

673. Wyke RJ, Edwards FC, Allan RN. Employment problems and prospects for patients with inflammatory bowel disease. *Gut* 1988; **29**: 346–51.

674. Travis SP. Review article: insurance risks for patients with ulcerative colitis or Crohn's disease. *Aliment Pharmacol Ther* 1997; **11**: 51–9.

675. Mayberry JF. The role of self-help groups for patients with inflammatory bowel disease. *Int J Colorectal Dis* 1987; **2**: 15–16.

676. Mayberry JF, Morris JS, Calcraft B et al. Information assessment by patients of a booklet on Crohn's disease. *Public Health* 1985; **99**: 239–42.

677. Dudley-Brown S. Prevention of psychological distress in persons with inflammatory bowel disease. *Issues Ment Health Nurs* 2002; **23**: 403–22.

678. Williams JG, Cheung WY, Russell IT et al. Open access follow up for inflammatory bowel disease: pragmatic randomised trial and cost effectiveness study. *Br Med J* 2000; **320**: 544–8.

679. Cheung WY, Dove J, Lervy B et al. Shared care in gastroenterology: GP's views of open access to out-patient follow-up for patients with inflammatory bowel disease. *Fam Pract* 2002; **19**: 53–6.

680. Anonymous. Inflammatory bowel disease. *MeReC Bull (Natl Prescribing Centre)* 1999; **10**: 45–8.

681. Robinson A, Thompson DG, Wilkin D et al. Guided self-management and patient-directed follow-up of ulcerative colitis: a randomised trial. *Lancet* 2001; **358**: 976–81.

682. Nightingale AJ. The IBD nurse: a key role in running the IBD service. In: Rampton DS, ed. *Inflammatory Bowel Disease, Clinical Diagnosis and Management*. London, UK: Martin Dunitz Ltd, 2000, 225–33.

683. Nightingale AJ, Middleton W, Middleton SJ et al. Evaluation of the effectiveness of a specialist nurse in the management of inflammatory bowel disease (IBD). *Eur J Gastroenterol Hepatol* 2000; **12**: 967–73.

684. Feagan BG. Review article: economic issues in Crohn's disease – assessing the effects of new treatments on health-related quality of life. *Aliment Pharmacol Ther* 1999; **13**(Suppl 4): 29–37.

685. Hanauer SB, Cohen RD, Becker RV III et al. Advances in the management of Crohn's disease: economics and clinical potential of infliximab. *Clin Ther* 1998; **20**: 1009–28.

686. Blomqvist P, Ekbom A. Inflammatory bowel diseases: health care and costs in Sweden in 1994. *Scand J Gastroenterol* 1997; **32**: 1134–9.

687. Hay AR, Hay JW. Inflammatory bowel disease: medical cost algorithms. *J Clin Gastroenterol* 1992; **14**: 318–27.
688. Hay JW, Hay AR. Inflammatory bowel disease: costs-of-illness. *J Clin Gastroenterol* 1992; **14**: 309–17.
689. Silverstein MD, Loftus EV, Sandborn WJ et al. Clinical course and costs of care for Crohn's disease: Markov model analysis of a population-based cohort. *Gastroenterology* 1999; **117**: 49–57.
690. Bernstein CN, Papineau N, Zajaczkowski J et al. Direct hospital costs for patients with inflammatory bowel disease in a Canadian tertiary care university hospital. *Am J Gastroenterol* 2000; **95**: 677–83.
691. Cohen RD, Larson LR, Roth JM et al. The cost of hospitalization in Crohn's disease. *Am J Gastroenterol* 2000; **95**: 524–30.
692. Blomqvist P, Feltelius N, Lofberg R et al. A 10-year survey of inflammatory bowel diseases – drug therapy, costs and adverse reactions. *Aliment Pharmacol Ther* 2001; **15**: 475–81.
693. Bonen DK, Cho JH. The genetics of inflammatory bowel disease. *Gastroenterology* 2003; **124**: 521–36.
694. Oberhuber G, Puspok A, Oesterreicher C et al. Focally enhanced gastritis: a frequent type of gastritis in patients with Crohn's disease. *Gastroenterology* 1997; **112**: 698–706.
695. Braun J, Brandt J, Listing J et al. Treatment of ankylosing spondylitis with infliximab: a randomised controlled multicentre trial. *Lancet* 2002; **359**: 1187–93.
696. Teahon K, Pearson M, Levi AJ et al. Elemental diet in the management of Crohn's disease during pregnancy. *Gut* 1991; **32**: 1079–81.
697. Schreiber S, Rutgeerts P, Fedorak R et al. CDP870, a humanized anti-TNF antibody fragment, induces clinical response with remission in patients with active Crohn's disease (CD). *Gastroenterology* 2003 (Abstr, in press).
698. den Broeder A, van de Putte L, Rau R et al. A single dose, placebo controlled study of the fully human anti-tumor necrosis factor-alpha antibody adalimumab (D2E7) in patients with rheumatoid arthritis. *J Rheumatol* 2002; **29**: 2288–98.

Appendix: addresses of patient support groups

United Kingdom and Ireland
National Association of Colitis and Crohn's disease (NACC)
4 Beaumont House
Sutton Road
St Albans
Hertfordshire AL1 5HH

Tel: 01727 844296 (information), 01727 830038 (administration)
Fax: 01727 862550
Website: http://www.nacc.org.uk
Email: nacc@nacc.org.uk

Ileostomy and Ileoanal Pouch Support Group (ia)
PO Box 132
Scunthorpe DN15 9YW

Tel: 01724 720150
Website: http://www.ileostomypouch.demon.co.uk
Email: ia@ileostomypouch.demon.co.uk

The Continence Foundation
307 Hatton Square
16 Baldwin Gardens,
London EC1N 7RJ

Tel: 020 7831 9831 (helpline), 020 7404 6875 (office)
Website: http://www.vois.org.uk/cf
Email: continence.foundation@dial.pipex.com

Digestive Disorders Foundation
3 St Andrews Place,
London NW1 4LB

Tel: 020 7486 0341
Fax: 020 7224 2012
Website: http://www.digestivedisorders.org.uk

Irish Society for Colitis and Crohn's Disease (ISCC)
Carmichael Centre
North Brunswick Street
Dublin-7
Ireland

Tel: +353 18721416
Fax: +353 18735737

Europe
European Federation of Crohn's and Ulcerative Colitis Associations (EFCCA)
c/o Tor Erik Jorgensen
Parallelen 13A
N-1430 As
Norway

Tel: +47 64941671
Fax: +47 22937213
Website: nacc.org.uk/efcca/
Email: efcca@hotmail.com

Rest of the world
Australian Crohn's and Colitis Association
PO Box 201
Moorolbark
VIC 3138
Australia

Tel: +61 (0)97269008

Canadian Foundation for Ileitis and Colitis
387 Bloor Street East
Suite 402
Toronto
Ontario M4W1H7
Canada

The Crohn's and Colitis Foundation of America
386 Park Avenue South
17th floor
New York NY 10016–8804
USA

Tel: +1 800 9322423/ +1 2126853440
Fax: +1 2127794098
Website: http://www.ccfa.org
Email: info@ccfa.org

South African Crohn's and Colitis Association
PO Box 2638
Cape Town 800
South Africa

Tel: +27 (0)21252350

Index

Note: CD = Crohn's disease

Coventry University